Clinicians' Guide to Asthma

Clinicians' Guide to Asthma

Kian Fan Chung MD DSc FRCP
Professor of Respiratory Medicine
National Heart & Lung Institute
Imperial College School of Medicine
and
Honorary Consultant Physician
Royal Brompton and Harefield NHS Trust
London

With a contribution by:

Andrew Bush MB BS (Hons) MA MD FRCP FRCPCH
Reader in Paediatric Respirology
National Heart & Lung Institute
Imperial College School of Medicine
and
Honorary Consultant Paediatric Chest Physician
Royal Brompton and Harefield NHS Trust
London

ARNOLD

A member of the Hodder Headline Group
LONDON · NEW YORK · NEW DELHI

First published in Great Britain in 2002 by
Arnold, a member of the Hodder Headline Group,
338 Euston Road, London NW1 3BH

http://www.arnoldpublishers.com

Distributed in the United States of America by
Oxford University Press Inc.,
198 Madison Avenue, New York, NY 10016
Oxford is a registered trademark of Oxford University Press

Whilst the advice and information in this book are believed to be true and
accurate at the date of going to press, neither the author[s] nor the publisher
can accept any legal responsibility or liability for any errors or omissions
that may be made. In particular (but without limiting the generality of the
preceding disclaimer) every effort has been made to check drug dosages;
however, it is still possible that errors have been missed. Furthermore,
dosage schedules are constantly being revised and new side-effects
recognized. For these reasons the reader is strongly urged to consult the
drug companies' printed instructions before administering any of the drugs
recommended in this book.

British Library Cataloguing in Publication Data
A catalogue record for this book is available from the British Library

Library of Congress Cataloging-in-Publication Data
A catalog record for this book is available from the Library of Congress

ISBN 0 340 76287 X

1 2 3 4 5 6 7 8 9 10

Commissioning Editor: Joanna Koster
Production Editor: Wendy Rooke
Production Controller: Iain McWilliams
Cover Designer: Terry Griffiths

Typeset in 11 on 13 pt Garamond by Charon Tec Pvt. Ltd, Chennai, India
Printed and bound in Malta by Gutenberg Press Ltd

What do you think about this book? Or any other Arnold title?
Please send your comments to feedback.arnold@hodder.co.uk

Contents

Preface   vii

List of abbreviations   viii

1. Definition, prevalence and impacts   1

2. Clinical diagnosis and assessment of asthma   13

3. Investigations and laboratory assessment of asthma   23

4. Mechanisms of asthma: risk factors and pathophysiology   39

5. Pharmacology and therapy of asthma   61

6. Management of chronic asthma and acute severe asthma   95

7. Asthma in infants and children   115
   Andrew Bush

8. Current and future challenge of asthma   135

Bibliography   147

Index   157

Preface

There is no doubt that asthma is one of the most common afflictions of industrialized countries and it is worrying that its prevalence is truly on the increase. Asthma also has a toll of morbidity and mortality. Some patients (thankfully only a minority) experience constant severe disruption to their lives, with recurrent exacerbations that can be life-threatening, and often with daily symptoms despite taking large amounts of medications. One of the most recent important events in the asthma world has been the setting up of national asthma guidelines for treating and combating the disease. More research continues on the causation and mechanism of the disease, and we have certainly learnt a lot over the past 10 years. The hope is that prevention, cure and better treatments will one day be available. In fact, I believe that significant advances may be on the horizon. My aim in writing this book has been to provide for the practising physician, or the novice researcher in asthma, an up-to-date account of what we know about asthma, in all its aspects. I also hope that the practising physician will find this book useful in the day-to-day management of asthma patients. I am extremely grateful to my colleague, Dr Andy Bush, for his contribution, the chapter on paediatric asthma, which fills in an important gap. I wish to thank Jo Koster and Peter Altman of Hodder for their utmost patience in allowing the project to go forward. My family has also been patient and I am deeply grateful for their understanding and support.

London
September 2001

List of abbreviations

AIRE	Asthma Insights and Reality in Europe
ALOX5	5-lipoxygenase
AP-1	(transcriptional) activator protein
APC	antigen-presenting cell
AQLQ	Asthma Quality of Life Questionnaire
BDP	beclomethasone dipropionate
BHR	bronchial hyperresponsiveness
BMP	beclomethasone monopropionate
BTS	British Thoracic Society
BUD	budesonide
cAMP	cyclic adenosine monophosphate
CCR	chemokine receptor
CFC	chlorofluorocarbon
COPD	chronic obstructive pulmonary disease
COX	cyclooxgenase
CT	computed tomography
cys-LT	cysteinyl-leukotriene
DPI	dry-powder inhaler
DSCG	disodium cromoglycate
ECP	eosinophil cationic protein
EDN	eosinophil-derived neurotoxin
EGF	epidermal growth factor
ELISA	enzyme-linked immunosorbent assay
eNO	exhaled nitric oxide
FEV_1	forced expiratory volume in the first second
FGF	fibroblast growth factor
FP	fluticasone propionate
FVC	forced vital capacity
GINA	Global Initiative for Asthma Management and Prevention
GM-CSF	granulocyte/macrophage colony stimulating factor
GR	glucocorticoid receptor
GRE	glucocorticoid receptor element
Gs	stimulatory G protein
HFC	hydrofluorocarbon
HIV	human immunodeficiency virus
ICAM	intercellular adhesion molecule
IFN	interferon
IgE	immunoglobulin E
IGF	insulin-like growth factor

IgG	immunoglobulin G
IL	interleukin
IL-4R	interleukin-4 receptor
iNOS	inducible nitric-oxide synthase
ISAAC	International Study of Asthma and Allergies in Childhood
LT	leukotriene
MCP	monocyte chemoattractant protein
MDI	metered-dose inhaler
MIP	macrophage inflammatory protein
MMEF	maximum mid-expiratory flow rate
NF-κB	nuclear factor-κB
NOS	nitric oxide synthase
PAF	platelet-activating factor
PC_{20}-FEV_1	the concentration of bronchoconstrictor agent (PC_{20}) needed to cause a 20% fall in FEV_1
PCR	polymerase chain reaction
PDGF	platelet-derived growth factor
PEFR	peak expiratory flow rate
PG	prostaglandin
pMDI	pressurized metered-dose inhaler
pMDI-SP	pressurized metered-dose inhaler with spacer
RANTES	regulated upon activation, normal T-cell expressed and secreted (achemokine)
RAST	radioallergosorbent test
RSV	respiratory syncytial virus
SCF	stem cell factor
STAT 6	signal transducer and activator of transcription 6
TF	transcription factor
TGF	transforming growth factor
Th	T-helper (cell)
Th0	undifferentiated T-helper (cell)
Th1	Th type 1
Th2	Th type 2
Thp	Th progenitor (cell)
TNF	tumour necrosis factor
VCAM	vascular cell adhesion molecule
VLA	very late antigen

Definition, prevalence and impacts

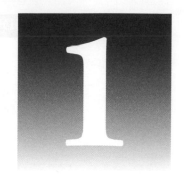

Definition

Since the first attempt was made in 1959, the condition termed 'asthma' has been difficult to define satisfactorily. There are many reasons for this. Asthma is such a heterogeneous condition, and we have a poor understanding of the causes, and of its natural history and pathophysiology. We also do not have a specific marker(s) for the disease. Several definitions have been put forward that describe the broad spectrum of the clinical phenotype, and in 1959, the definition focused on differentiating asthma from other chronic airway obstructive disorders, particularly emphysema and chronic bronchitis. With the passage of time, the definition of asthma has evolved and this can be approached from several angles:

- clinical: a combination of symptoms (intermittent wheeze, cough and shortness of breath);
- lung function tests showing variability of airflow obstruction (peak expiratory flow rate diurnal variability with asthma exacerbation);
- bronchial hyperresponsiveness as a shift of the concentration–FEV_1 (forced expiratory volume in the first second) curve to the left, with an increased plateau response;
- airway inflammation with bronchial mucosal infiltration with inflammatory cells, such as eosinophils and T cells.

CLINICAL PRESENTATION

For the clinician, the diagnosis of asthma is not difficult in most cases where this is made on the basis of the history and on the response to specific treatments. He or she recognizes bronchial asthma as being recurrent episodes of airflow limitation that are usually reversible. The symptoms consist of breathlessness, wheezing, chest tightness and cough, sometimes productive of sputum. While these symptoms may be reversible spontaneously, more often they respond quickly to bronchodilators, in particular inhaled β-adrenergic agonists. Anatomically, asthma affects both the central and more distal airways.

Symptoms of airflow obstruction are variable with time, and there may be more severe episodes that need urgent medical attention (exacerbations). The outcome is variable, with death during an exacerbation if untreated, or resolution of symptoms within a short period of time, or the development of chronic airflow limitation over the years.

MEASUREMENT OF LUNG FUNCTION

The presence or absence of airways obstruction itself is not an important factor in the diagnosis of asthma, although it provides an index of the severity of asthma in an already diagnosed patient. The ability to measure peak flow rates at regular intervals has led to the observation that asthmatics may have an excessive diurnal variation of airflow obstruction, usually in the early morning, as often characterized by the early morning wheeze. Measurement of lung function to assess the airways response to inhaled bronchodilators, such as β-adrenergic agonists, has also been useful to establish what a significant degree of reversibility is for inclusion in any definition of asthma. For FEV_1, for example, an improvement of 15–20 per cent is considered significant enough to support a diagnosis of asthma.

BRONCHIAL HYPERRESPONSIVENESS

One of the earlier findings regarding asthma is the abnormal response of the airways to a provoking bronchoconstrictor stimulus, such as inhaled methacholine or histamine, or exercise. The asthmatic individual shows a greater degree of responsiveness than the non-asthmatic individual, in terms of a smaller amount of bronchoconstrictor agent causing a similar degree of bronchoconstriction, or of the maximal degree of worsening of lung function. Such measurements may be abnormal even in asymptomatic asthmatics, and are so characteristic in asthma patients that this has been included within the definition of asthma. Although other airway obstructive conditions, such as chronic obstructive pulmonary disease, do share bronchial hyperresponsiveness (BHR), the degree of BHR is usually mild. However, the presence of BHR in the absence of symptoms is not considered to be asthma, although this is a predisposing factor to the onset of asthma. Some workers consider the degree of BHR as indicative of the severity of asthma. The causes of BHR are not known, but may include airway wall thickening, airway inflammation and/or abnormal airway smooth muscle contractility.

AIRWAY INFLAMMATION

The definition of asthma has been particularly enhanced by the recognition over the past 20 years that the airways submucosa of patients with asthma is chronically inflamed with a cellular infiltrate characterized by eosinophils and T cells, together with epithelial damage and fragility. Often, there is subepithelial fibrosis characterized by an increased thickness of the 'basement membrane'. This characteristic inflammatory response could be used to separate asthma from other airway conditions, such as chronic obstructive pulmonary disease and emphysema, which often cause diagnostic confusion with asthma. The inflammatory process is presumed to cause the main characteristics of airways obstruction and bronchial hyperresponsiveness, but how this inflammatory process starts remains elusive. While reversibility of airflow obstruction, spontaneously or by pharmacological means, is an important component of asthma, airflow obstruction is not always totally reversible, and, indeed, there may be total loss of reversibility of airways obstruction resulting from the chronic inflammatory process.

DEFINITION OF ASTHMA

The definition of asthma remains clinically based but backed by the use of physiological measurements, by the response of the airways to pharmacological agents and by the presence of specific pathological changes. One such definition comes from the British Thoracic Guidelines published in 1988, and encompasses all the major points raised above:

> Asthma is a common and chronic inflammatory condition of the airways whose cause is not completely understood. As a result of inflammation the airways are hyperresponsive and they narrow easily in response to a wide range of stimuli. This may result in coughing, wheezing, chest tightness, and shortness of breath and these symptoms are often worse at night. Narrowing of the airways is usually reversible, but in some patients with chronic asthma the inflammation may lead to irreversible airflow obstruction. Characteristic pathological features include the presence in the airway of inflammatory cells, plasma exudation, oedema, smooth muscle hypertrophy, mucus plugging, and shedding of the epithelium.

Given our current understanding of the pathophysiology of asthma, this is the best definition available, because it attempts to encompass most of the clinical phenotypes of asthma. What the definition does not include are the cut-off points for the various parameters that are needed to define asthma, such as the degree of reversibility or the amount of inflammation. In reporting research studies, it is important to define the criteria by which patients with asthma have been recruited.

Epidemiology of asthma

PREVALENCE STUDIES

Asthma is one of the most common chronic disease worldwide. Prevalence studies have been performed by asking for a history of intermittent wheeze.

Standardized and validated methods to document the prevalence of asthma have shown large degrees of variation in the world. In the International Study of Asthma and Allergies in Childhood (ISAAC) of half a million children aged 6–7 years and 13–14 years in 56 countries, the prevalence of wheeze in the year prior to the survey varied from 6 to 32 per cent and from 2 to 33 per cent, respectively (Figure 1.1). The prevalence was highest in the affluent English-speaking countries, intermediate in western Europe, Latin America, Africa and South-East Asia, and lowest in India, China, eastern Europe and

Figure 1.1
Worldwide variation in prevalence of self-reported symptoms of asthma in response to written questionnaires amongst schoolchildren aged 13–14 years in various countries. (From the International Study of Asthma and Allergies in Childhood (ISAAC) study (1998), reprinted with permission from Elsevier Science from *The Lancet*, 1998, **351**, 1225–32.)

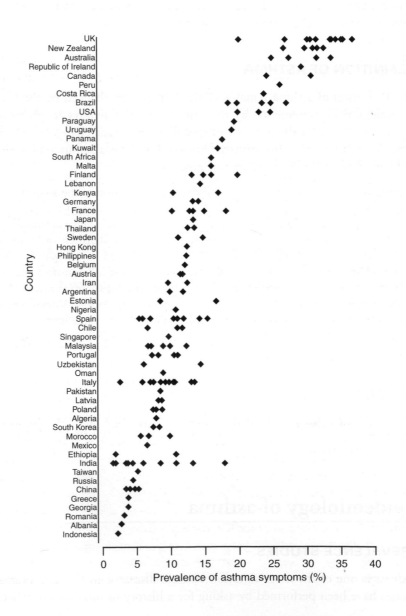

the former Soviet Union. There was a correlation between the rates of asthma with those of rhinoconjunctivitis.

A wide geographic variation in the prevalence of physician-diagnosed asthma has been reported in Europe, with the highest prevalence in the UK and in some centres in France, and the lowest prevalence in East Germany and Spain. The geographical variation in atopic sensitization corresponded closely to the geographical variation of asthma. The prevalence of physician-diagnosed asthma correlated well with the use of anti-asthma medication. There is little variation in asthma prevalence among children or adults throughout the UK. The reported inter-country variation is the result of many factors, including environmental factors and differences in treatment practices.

In the ISAAC study of 12–14-year-olds in a large sample of mixed secondary schools across Great Britain, almost 1 in 5 had used asthma treatment in the past year, and 21 per cent reported ever having a diagnosis of asthma. One estimate is that 3.4 million people in the UK – 1 out of every 7 children aged between 2 and 15 years (1.5 million) and 1 out of every 25 adults (1.9 million) – have asthma symptoms requiring treatment. One worrying feature about the prevalence of asthma is the increase in many countries, such as the UK, over recent decades. In a survey conducted in Leicester, asthma and wheezing in children under 5 years has almost doubled in less than a decade, with 11.6 per cent children in 1990 and 21.3 per cent in 1998 diagnosed as having asthma. Over 30 years in Aberdeen, parental awareness of doctor-diagnosed asthma had increased from 4.1 to 18.7 per cent. This recent increase in prevalence of asthma was accompanied by a more than twofold increase in visits to general practitioners' surgeries because of asthma between 1981/82 and 1991/92, with the number of people consulting for asthma for the first time having more than tripled. This increase in prevalence is not likely to be due to the condition being more recognized by parents, patients or doctors.

SEVERITY OF ASTHMA

The severity of asthma can be defined in many ways, including: the frequency of daily symptoms; the need for medical consultations, either at the surgery or attendance in casualty departments; time taken off work or school and a poor quality of life characterized by non-participation in communal activities such as sports. Other parameters that can define the severity of asthma include: the number of admissions to hospital for treatment of acute severe asthma episodes; the variability in peak flow measurements and lung function tests. More recently, quality-of-life scores and socioeconomic considerations have been used. Random survey questionnaires or telephone interviews have usually been used in assessing the impact of asthma in the community.

Such surveys invoke a picture of continuing asthma symptoms. In a 1996 health survey for England, of those adults who had experienced wheezing in the past 12 months, 19 per cent had their sleep disturbed once or more a week, and 50 per cent had symptoms that interfered with their daily activities. In 1996, 11 per cent of adults and 19 per cent of children had been admitted to hospital on at least one occasion because of their asthma, amounting to 85 287 admissions to hospital, and the average length of stay in hospital for asthma was 3.2 days. Over one-third of children with asthma miss more than 1 week from school per year and up to 49 per cent of working adults had time off work because of asthma, with 9 per cent not able to work at all. In a survey of 785 asthmatics by the UK National Asthma Campaign, up to 34 per cent were experiencing significant consequences of their asthma, having been classified as having moderately severe or severe asthma.

Asthma is a continuing problem and concern in a significant proportion of patients, and this is even observed in patients who are taking asthma treatment. In a telephone survey carried out across Europe in 1999 (AIRE: Asthma insights and reality in Europe), 30 per cent of patients said that they had been disturbed by their asthma during sleep over the past week, 63 per cent had some form of daily living activities limited by their asthma, 61 per cent experienced severe episodes of coughing, wheezing, chest tightness or shortness of breath, and 30 per cent had emergency visits to hospital or doctor in the past year. Yet, in this sample, 41 per cent of patients reported that they were being treated with a prescription medication to reduce or prevent asthma. This survey indicates that there may be problems related to the delivery of asthma care and possibly problems with patients taking their medication.

MORTALITY FROM ASTHMA

Asthma mortality is generally low, although there have been increases in asthma mortality during certain periods, such as the increase between 1964 and 1966 in England and Wales, Australia and New Zealand, and the increase between 1977 and 1983 in New Zealand. There has been a gradual trend in increased asthma mortality in the UK, Canada and the USA between 1974 and 1985, with a doubling of the mortality rate over that period in the latter two countries. However, in the UK, after the peak in the late 1980s, at 39 deaths per million of the population, there has been a gradual decline, to 27 deaths per million in 1997 (the number of deaths attributed to asthma being 1584 out of a total of 63 000 deaths in the UK, i.e. a 2.5 per cent mortality rate). In England and Wales, asthma mortality is now falling by approximately 6 per cent each year in people aged 5–64 years (Figure 1.2).

Can we prevent asthma deaths? Many risk factors for asthma deaths have been identified in retrospective studies of asthma mortality. These include age

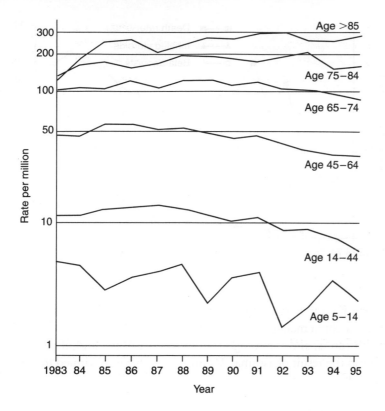

Figure 1.2
Asthma deaths per million population subdivided into various age groups from 1983 to 1995 in England and Wales, demonstrating the trend towards a reduction in asthma deaths. (Reproduced with permission of the BMJ Publishing Group Campbell *et al.* (1997) *BMJ* **314**, 1439–41.)

(for those over 40 years), cigarette smoking, ethnicity, psychosocial factors, a past history of severe or life-threatening attacks, previous hospital admissions and emergency room visits, and discontinuity of physician care. A fatal outcome was also associated with inadequate assessment and inappropriate treatment of severe asthma, with overreliance on high doses of bronchodilator therapy and insufficient use of corticosteroids. In the more labile and atopic patient, eosinophilia and a greater degree of reversibility were recognized as risk factors.

Use of excessive isoproterenol has been blamed for the increased asthma deaths that occurred in the period 1964–66, and increased prescriptions for the short-acting β_2-agonist, fenoterol, have been associated with a greater risk of mortality in the asthma epidemic in New Zealand in the 1980s. Effective withdrawal of fenoterol from the market in New Zealand was followed by a fall in asthma mortality, although some of this reduction may also have been due to a greater use of anti-inflammatory therapy, in particular inhaled corticosteroids (Figure 1.3). Overreliance on β-agonists may be a direct or indirect risk factor and may have served as a marker of severe asthma requiring urgent action, thus underlying the fall in asthma mortality. The gradual reduction in mortality in the UK over the past decade may have been due to a combination of factors, including: increased use of inhaled corticosteroids, reduced reliance

Figure 1.3
Asthma deaths per
100 000 in New Zealand
between 1973 and 1992,
and prescriptions of
β-agonists and inhaled
corticosteroids in
millions of doses.
(R Beasley, N Pearce
et al, "Asthma mortality
and inhaled beta agonist
therapy", *Australian and
New Zealand Journal of
Medicine.* (1991) Vol 21:
753–763. Figure 1.3,
reproduced with
permission.)

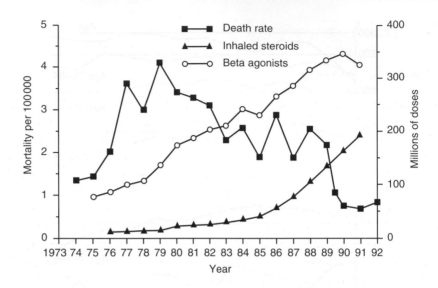

on potent β_2-adrenergic agonists, better education of patients (and doctors) regarding asthma management, adherence to national management guidelines by health carers, and the recognition of severe asthma and of patients at risk of dying as the result of asthma. Asthma deaths have continued to fall over the past 5 years.

HEALTH ECONOMICS

There is a paucity of studies of the economic impacts of asthma. Most studies provide an overall estimate of the medical and indirect costs associated with asthma. Costs related to asthma can be divided into costs to the health service, and the indirect costs to the community caused by loss of productivity. The rising costs with the introduction of new drug therapies highlight the need for accurate evaluation of the health economics of asthma. Such information may be used to justify the use and expense of new therapies to control asthma, and may also provide a better measure of the impact that asthma has on the community.

In 1995/96, asthma was estimated to have cost the National Health Service £672 million, with £60 million being the cost of primary-care consultations, £511 million for prescription of drugs, £50 million for the costs of hospital admissions due to asthma and £5.5 million for outpatient management. Other costs of asthma include Department of Social Security sickness invalidity benefits, estimated at £161 million, and a reduction in productivity estimated at £1226 million based on 18.3 million days' incapacity due to asthma. Therefore, the total costs were estimated to be over £2 billion in 1995/96.

Natural history

EARLY CHILDHOOD

The incidence of asthma is highest in early childhood, decreasing throughout later childhood and adolescence. In a cohort study from Tucson, Arizona, USA, which examined the development and persistence of asthma in the first 6 years of life, 34 per cent of children developed asthma during the first 3 years of life, and a further 15 per cent developed wheezing between 3 and 6 years of age. Among the 34 per cent that developed wheezing symptoms before the age of 3, 20 per cent were symptom-free by the age of 6 years, while the remaining 14 per cent had persistent wheezing. Therefore, the majority of wheezers had remitted. The persistent wheezers at age 6 more often had a family history of asthma (particularly maternal), elevated immunoglobulin E (IgE) levels in infancy and at age 6 years, and had decreased lung function at age 6 but not in the first year of life.

The evolution of childhood asthma into adulthood has been studied in several longitudinal studies because few studies provide information on the incidence and long-term outcome of chronic asthma and wheezing during the school years. However, most studies indicate that in some patients there is disease remission, while in others there is persistence of symptoms, ranging from mild to severe in extent. Between 30 and 70 per cent of children with asthma become markedly improved or symptom-free by early adulthood, but significant asthma symptoms persist in about 30 per cent. Some may have asymptomatic periods before developing wheeze again as adults.

In an Australian study that followed children from 7 to 35 years of age, wheezing episodes that started after the age of 3 years were usually associated with viral infections, and were rarely troublesome. Of children in this group, 40–50 per cent had no episodes by age 10, with continuing remission into adolescence. Ten to 20 per cent of children who had remission of symptoms by age 10 relapsed by adolescence or early adulthood. In the other group of children, who started to wheeze before the age of 3 years, early onset symptoms were characteristic of children who later developed chronic asthma that persisted during childhood and into adult life. The most troublesome period was observed between the ages of 8 and 14, with airway obstruction being persistent over months. These asthmatics were usually male and had very hyperresponsive airways. Sixty per cent of these continued to have persistent and troublesome symptoms into adulthood associated with lower lung function.

In a cohort of UK children reviewed between birth and age 33 years on several occasions, the prevalence of asthma or wheeze over the past 12 months at ages 7, 11, 16 and 23 were 8, 5, 3 and 4 per cent. At age 7, there was a 50 per cent remission of early childhood wheeze, compared to 18, 10 and

10 per cent at ages 11, 16 and 23; however, there was a significant relapse rate, with 27 per cent prevalence of symptoms, at age 33.

What are the features that are associated with persistence of childhood asthma? Significant deterioration of lung function by age 6 appears to be a predictor of persistent wheeze. As to the persistence of childhood asthma, the following factors have been implicated: a family history of asthma, particularly maternal; an allergic background, particularly house dust mite sensitivity; maternal smoking; and the severity of childhood asthma, as judged by lung function, bronchial responsiveness or frequency of asthma episodes. Sensitization and exposure to house dust mite (and cockroaches, as found in some inner cities in the US) is very common amongst children and young adults attending emergency rooms for treatment of severe asthma episodes. Children with mild asthma are likely to have a good prognosis, but children with moderate or severe asthma will likely continue to have some degree of airway hyperresponsiveness and will be at risk from the long-term effects of asthma throughout life.

ADULT ASTHMA

Asthma can also begin in adulthood. Sometimes this may be in response to sensitizing agents in the workplace leading to occupational asthma, or from the development of atopy later in life, or it may not be associated with an atopic background at all. Often, there is a history of an upper respiratory tract viral infection with the first exacerbation. Occasionally this is seen in a patient

Figure 1.4
Changes with age in forced expiratory volume in one second (FEV_1) according to sex and the presence or absence of asthma. Asthmatics show a more rapid decline in FEV_1 than non-asthmatics. (Reproduced by permission from Lange *et al.* (1998) *N. Engl. J. Med.* **339**, 1194–2000. Copyright © 1998 Massachusetts Medical Society.)

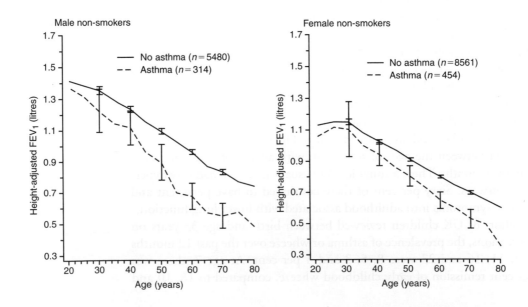

who has had childhood asthma that remitted in adolescence. In a study of adult asthma in Tucson, Arizona, USA, the change in prevalence over an 8-year period was small, and remission was uncommon. Remission of adult asthma was confirmed to be rare in other studies. In occupational asthma, asthmatics may have persistent symptoms, with abnormal pulmonary function tests and bronchial hyperresponsiveness, despite removal from exposure. Irreversible airflow obstruction may develop in adult asthma in the absence of smoking, particularly in those over 65 years. Asthmatics experience a more rapid decline in the lung function measurement of FEV_1 than non-asthmatics, and smoking asthmatics have the greatest decline in FEV_1 (Figure 1.4). There are correlations between the severity of lung function, airway hyperresponsiveness, bronchodilator response to β-agonists, mucus hypersecretion and cigarette smoking.

Clinical diagnosis and assessment of asthma

The diagnosis and assessment of asthma are based on the patient's medical history, physical examination and laboratory investigations. The common clinical features of asthma are recurrent episodes of wheezing, chest tightness, cough and shortness of breath. Asthmatic patients present with a spectrum of signs and symptoms that vary in degree of severity from patient to patient and within the same patient over time. In addition, some patients, particularly the elderly, may be poor perceivers of airways obstruction.

Paroxysmal episodes may be provoked by allergic stimuli, such as exposure to an allergen to which the asthmatic is sensitive. Some cases of asthma may be entirely seasonal, such as pollen-induced asthma in the summer months. Non-pulmonary symptoms that indicate the presence of allergies, such as rhinitis, conjunctivitis and eczema, are common in such patients. Non-allergic stimuli, such as cold air, exercise, common upper respiratory tract viral infections and irritants, may also provoke symptoms. Some asthmatics develop exacerbations of their asthma when taking aspirin and other non-steroidal anti-inflammatory drugs. Occupational asthma, induced by specific chemicals or proteins encountered at the workplace following sensitization, may also present in relation to exposure at work. A list of trigger factors for asthma is shown in Box 2.1.

Severe episodes of asthma may occur very rapidly, sometimes over a period of a few minutes ('brittle asthma'), and may be life threatening. Asthma may also present with chronic persistent symptoms, often characterized by worsening symptoms at night or on waking in the mornings. These patients often develop asthma later on in life, and have concomitant rhinosinusitis and nasal polyps.

Questionnaires have been used to diagnose and assess asthma, on the basis of symptoms, for epidemiological studies. One such questionnaire, developed by the International Union Against Tuberculosis and Lung Diseases (IUATLD), included the following questions:

1. Have you had wheezing or whistling in your chest in the last 12 months?
2. Have you had an attack of wheezing that came after stopping exercise?
3. Have you woken up with an attack of wheezing at any time?

Box 2.1
Triggers of asthma

- Common viral infections of upper respiratory tract
- Aeroallergens such as house dust mite, pollens, animal danders
- Occupational agents such as isocyanates, epoxyresins, laboratory animals, flour
- Exercise
- Cold air
- Hyperventilation
- Water, hypotonic and hypertonic aerosols
- Drugs, such as aspirin and non-steroidal anti-inflammatory drugs, β-adrenergic blockers
- Foods and drinks, such as nuts, milk and egg allergies; preservatives, such as metabisulphite; or colouring agents, such as tartrazine
- Gastro-oesophageal reflux
- Environmental pollutants, such as traffic fumes; irritants, such as cigarette smoke
- Psychological factors (may relate to hyperventilation)

4. Have you woken up with an attack of cough at any time?
5. Have you had an attack of shortness of breath that came during the day when you were at rest at any time?
6. Have you had a feeling of chest tightness on waking in the morning?
7. Have you had an attack of asthma?

The questions that predicted asthma the best were those that asked about wheeze at rest or following exercise, asthma attack, chest tightness and shortness of breath at rest.

Underdiagnosis of asthma in both children and adults has been reported as a frequent problem. The diagnosis may not be made because of the non-specific nature of asthma symptoms or because the patients may tolerate intermittent respiratory symptoms of wheeze and chest tightness before obtaining a medical opinion, or may be poor perceivers of their disabilities or symptoms. Children who wheeze only when they have respiratory infections may be dismissed as wheezy bronchitis or pneumonia.

A comprehensive list of questions making up the medical history of asthma is shown in Box 2.2.

1. Symptoms:
   (a) cough, wheeze, shortness of breath, chest tightness and sputum production
   (b) conditions associated with asthma: rhinitis, sinusitis, nasal polyposis, atopic dermatitis.
2. Pattern of symptoms:
   (a) perennial, seasonal, or perennial with seasonal exacerbations
   (b) continuous, episodic or both
   (c) onset, duration and frequency of symptoms
   (d) diurnal variation of symptoms; nocturnal symptoms.
3. Precipitating or aggravating factors:
   (a) upper respiratory viral infections
   (b) exposure to environmental allergens: house dust mite, pollens, animal fur (cat and dogs)
   (c) exposure to occupational chemicals or allergens (including animal urine or saliva)
   (d) exposure to irritants, tobacco smoke, air pollutants, chemicals, etc.
   (e) influence of emotional states and stress
   (f) drugs: aspirin or non-steroidal anti-inflammatory agents, beta-blockers (including eye drops)
   (g) exercise
   (h) change in weather conditions
   (i) endocrine factors: menstrual periods, pregnancy, thyroid disease.
4. History of disease development:
   (a) age of onset/diagnosis
   (b) evolution of disease
   (c) previous and current management of disease and response to treatment.
5. Profile of exacerbation: speed of attack, management and outcome.
6. Social situation; housing condition: exposure to indoor allergens, animals at home, exposure to cigarette smoke, dampness, heating.
7. Severity of disease:
   (a) number of emergency treatments, including admissions to hospital or courses of oral corticosteroids
   (b) number of life-threatening episodes
   (c) number of school or work days missed
   (d) limitation of activity (e.g. sports)
   (e) frequency of nocturnal awakenings
   (f) effect on growth, behaviour, school or work achievements.
8. Impact of disease on family and relatives.
9. Family history: asthma or allergies in close relatives.

Box 2.2
Medical history for asthma

Physical examination

The physical examination is helpful in the diagnosis if signs of airflow obstruction are present at the time of examination. Analysis of these signs can give an accurate picture of the severity of asthma. Airflow obstruction secondary to airway smooth muscle contraction, airway oedema and mucus hypersecretion leads to the patient breathing at a higher lung volume to increase outward retraction of the airways, in an attempt to maintain their patency. The combination of hyperinflation and severe airflow obstruction found during an asthma exacerbation increases the work of breathing. Expiratory wheeze is the typical sign of airflow limitation caused by airflow turbulence, but is not a sensitive marker of airways obstruction. Wheezing may disappear with increasing severity of an asthma exacerbation when the patient is too weak to generate enough airflow turbulence in his very narrowed airways. Other signs of worsening asthma include inability to speak in complete sentences, hyperinflated chest, use of accessory muscles of respiration with intercostal recession, and pulsus paradoxus of greater than 15 mm of mercury pressure; cyanosis and drowsiness may appear. Occasionally, in acute severe asthma, there may be evidence of lobar collapse due to mucus plugging of the large airways.

Varying degrees of severity of acute asthma may present as follows:

1. Mild to moderate: wheezing or coughing without severe distress, able to hold conversation normally, some degree of shortness of breath, peak flow likely to be within 50 per cent of best value.
2. Moderate to severe: wheezing or coughing with some distress, talking in short sentences or phrases, breathing rate increased and tachycardia, peak flow usually less than 50 per cent predicted, some degree of oxygen desaturation (90–95 per cent).
3. Severe, life-threatening: severe respiratory distress, difficulty in talking, cyanosis of tongue, tired and confused, poor respiratory effort with few wheezes ('silent chest') and weak breath sounds, tachypnoea, bradycardia and hypotension, peak flow less than 30 per cent predicted, oxygen saturation of less than 90 per cent.

Differential diagnosis

Although recurrent episodes of cough and wheeze are almost always due to asthma in children and adults, one must be aware that there are other rarer causes of airways obstruction that can cause similar symptoms and signs (Box 2.3). One needs a degree of suspicion, to take a careful history and examination to detect any particular unusual features, and be ready to investigate.

- Chronic obstructive pulmonary disease (COPD)
- Emphysema
- Chronic inflammatory airways disease (e.g. bronchiectasis, cystic fibrosis, bronchiolitis)
- Congestive cardiac failure ('cardiac asthma')
- Central airway obstruction caused by intraluminal tumour or by external compression
- Aspiration of foreign body
- Pulmonary embolism
- Carcinoid syndrome
- Extrinsic allergic alveolitis
- Eosinophilic pneumonitis: Churg–Strauss syndrome; allergic bronchopulmonary aspergillosis
- Sarcoidosis
- Vocal cord dysfunction
- Psychological factors
- Factitious asthma
- Causes of chronic cough

Box 2.3
Differential diagnosis of asthma

One of the potentially confusing symptom in terms of diagnosis of asthma is cough. A cough, particularly occurring at night, may or may not be accompanied by wheeze, and this has been classified as 'cough variant' asthma, particularly in children who may present with features associated with asthma, such as bronchial hyperresponsiveness, increased diurnal variation in peak flow measurements, and evidence of allergies; the cough usually responds well to inhaled corticosteroid therapy. However, if the cough does not have these features, other diagnoses that may be associated with the cough should be sought (e.g. post-nasal drip, gastro-oesophageal reflux or chronic bronchitis). A condition of eosinophilic bronchitis presenting with a chronic cough productive of eosinophils, and responding well to corticosteroids, has also been described. There are no particular features of asthma.

CHRONIC OBSTRUCTIVE PULMONARY DISEASE

Differentiating between asthma and chronic obstructive pulmonary disease (COPD) and emphysema, which is largely secondary to cigarette smoking, can be difficult. COPD is a progressive condition of airflow obstruction due to obstruction of the small airways associated with inflammation, and emphysema is the permanent destruction of alveolar walls with permanent enlargement of airspaces. There may be accompanying chronic bronchitis, with a chronic cough and sputum production. Asthma and COPD may coexist (often the term 'asthmatic bronchitis' is used) and asthma may manifest itself at any age. It is often difficult to ascertain the exact category in a particular smoker patient presenting with cough, shortness of breath and wheeze, although the intractable symptoms on exertion and lack of diurnal variability of symptoms or of airflow obstruction may point towards the 'fixed' airways obstruction of COPD. However, chronic long-standing asthma may also become 'fixed'. Often a corticosteroid trial (e.g. prednisolone 40 mg/day administered orally for 2 weeks) that results in a significant improvement in airflow obstruction is taken as evidence of asthma. Other pointers towards asthma may include significant diurnal variation of peak flow and eosinophilia in peripheral blood or in sputum. Lung function tests may show relatively fixed obstructive defect associated with a decreased diffusing capacity, which would favour the presence of COPD with emphysema, while thin-section computed tomography (CT) scans may provide a quantification of emphysema. The presence of eosinophils in sputum may point towards asthma and a beneficial response of the airflow obstruction to corticosteroid therapy. It is important to make the distinction, since management of certain aspects of these conditions may be different.

PAROXYSMAL NOCTURNAL DYSPNOEA

Congestive cardiac failure often presents with acute episodes of nocturnal dyspnoea with wheeze, often referred to as cardiac asthma. Distinction from asthma may be made by the concomitant clinical and radiological features of congestive cardiac failure, and usually relief of shortness of breath on assuming the upright position, although use of a β-agonist inhaler may also lead to relief of symptoms of wheeze and breathlessness. Paroxysmal nocturnal dyspnoea and asthma may coexist in some patients. Patients with bronchial asthma or COPD may develop left heart failure that presents clinically as exacerbation of wheezing and dyspnoea.

CENTRAL AIRWAY OBSTRUCTION

Partial obstruction of the central airways, such as the pharynx, larynx, trachea and both main bronchi, may result in symptoms that are similar to those of asthma. Other features that may indicate a central airway obstruction include inspiratory stridor, brassy cough, hoarseness, a mass in the neck and chest pain, associated with a poor response to asthma therapy. There are many potential causes of central airway obstruction, including: extrinsic tracheal compression, such as mediastinal tumours; intramural tracheal disease, such as stricture or tracheomalacia; and intraluminal tracheal disease, such as tumours and foreign bodies. Lung function test may reveal marked reduction in both expiratory and inspiratory flows, indicating a fixed central obstruction, while inspiratory or expiratory flow limitation may occur alone, dependent on the extrathoracic or intrathoracic site of the obstruction, respectively.

OTHER CONDITIONS

A carcinoid tumour may induce wheeze if present as an intraluminal tumour of the central airways, but this can also be induced in the carcinoid syndrome by the release of vasoactive and bronchoconstrictor substances, such as serotonin, in the circulation. Pulmonary embolism may also present with wheeze, from the release of constrictor mediators during the embolism. Sarcoidosis involving the larger airways endobronchially may cause intraluminal narrowing and wheeze and shortness of breath.

VOCAL CORD DYSFUNCTION

Vocal cord dysfunction is an important differential diagnosis in young patients in whom there are episodes of semiclosure of the glottis, producing both inspiratory and expiratory wheezes, often best heard at the open mouth or over the larynx, and being fainter in the lung fields. There may be surrounding circumstances of psychiatric illness or psychological stress. Usually, there is marked variability and lability of symptoms and signs, normal blood gases during episodes, normal lung function tests and poor response to asthma treatments. Sometimes, at indirect laryngoscopic examination, closure of the glottis can be observed.

It is important to note that there is sometimes associated vocal cord dysfunction during a genuine episode of asthma exacerbation. Therefore, these patients should not be labelled as having psychogenic asthma.

CHURG–STRAUSS SYNDROME

Churg–Strauss syndrome is an unusual disease, characterized by allergic granulomatosis and angiitis. It consists of an initial phase of asthma associated with a very marked blood eosinophilia and eosinophilic vasculitis. This gives rise to pulmonary infiltrates, myocarditis, myositis, neuritis, skin nodules and rashes, and glomerulonephritis. The condition usually responds rapidly to corticosteroids, although the recommended treatment is cyclophosphamide and corticosteroids. Recently, several cases of Churg–Strauss syndrome have been diagnosed in asthmatic patients given the leukotriene antagonists, zafirlukast or montelukast. It is not clear whether this is an unmasking of Churg–Strauss syndrome while oral corticosteroid treatment was being curtailed or whether this is a direct effect of these leukotriene antagonists.

ALLERGIC BRONCHOPULMONARY ASPERGILLOSIS

Patients with asthma may develop an allergic reaction to the fungus, *Aspergillus fumigatus*. They demonstrate precipitating antibodies to aspergillus in their serum, and positive skin-prick tests to this allergen. Some patients develop bronchopulmonary aspergillosis in which there is bronchial inflammation with eosinophils, and high levels of IgE in the blood. There may be eosinophilic infiltrates in the lung, observed as fleeting shadows on the chest radiograph. There is obstruction of the bronchi by mucus plugs and the persistent eosinophilic inflammation leads to bronchiectasis, usually seen in the proximal bronchi. Treatment usually consists of oral and inhaled corticosteroids to dampen down the intense airway inflammatory response that leads to airway wall damage.

Referral of patients to a specialist asthma clinic

Most patients with asthma can be diagnosed and managed well in general practice, but particular patients may benefit from specialist care from a chest physician. A suggested list of indications for such referrals is:

1. patients with uncontrolled, severe, life-threatening asthma;
2. patients with difficult-to-control asthma despite apparently adequate therapy;
3. patients in whom there may be a diagnostic problem, e.g. differentiation of asthma from chronic obstructive pulmonary disease in adults, chronic cough or cystic fibrosis in children;
4. presence of associated aggravating factors, such as sinus disease, rhinitis, nasal polyps and bronchopulmonary aspergillosis;
5. suspicion of occupational factors aggravating or causing asthma;
6. patients needing advice on environmental control, allergen avoidance, smoking cessation or on adherence to therapy.

Different clinical presentations of asthma and asthma severity

Given the varied presentation and course of the disease, it is not surprising that asthma has been grouped in various ways, such as on the basis of provoking factors, of severity, of pattern of asthma attacks and even on response to available treatments (Box 2.4). There is as yet no good classification on the basis of underlying basic mechanisms, since there is currently poor understanding of these mechanisms. This raises the important question as to whether there are different phenotypes of asthma, or whether there is only

Box 2.4
Different types of
asthma

- Atopic or non-atopic asthma
- Early onset (childhood) or late onset (adult) asthma
- Nocturnal asthma
- Exercise-induced asthma
- Aspirin-induced asthma
- Occupational asthma
- Seasonal asthma
- Cough variant asthma
- Acute severe asthma
- Chronic severe asthma
- Asthma deaths
- 'Fixed' irreversible asthma
- 'Brittle' asthma
- Corticosteroid resistant asthma
- Corticosteroid dependent asthma
- Churg–Strauss syndrome
- Allergic bronchopulmonary aspergillosis

one central mechanism, with varying severity of disease and interactions with exogenous factors to create such a varied presentation and course. Although there is no scientific rationale for classifying asthma according to Box 2.4, this is, nevertheless, useful as a starting point to define patient populations for analysis of mechanisms or of genetic abnormalities.

Classification according to severity is most useful to the clinician, since this could be used to gauge the amount and type of treatment needed to control asthma, both in the short and long term. Levels of severity of asthma can be described according to symptoms, as well as according to objective measurements of lung function and to the diurnal variability of peak flows. Surprisingly, there is no satisfactory scale of an overall integrated measure of symptoms for asthma. Specific quality-of-life questionnaires have been developed to reflect the impact of the chronic disease, not only on daily activities but also on psychological impairment. They may be used as a measure of severity. One of the problems with the classification of asthma severity is that the condition can vary from day to day, and often goes into periods of remission. One possibility for overcoming this variability is to describe severity over a short period (e.g. over the immediate previous month: 'activity') and also over the immediate past year (as a summation of the last 12 months: 'severity'). Descriptive terms have been used to indicate severity, such as persistent asthma,

Asthma severity	Symptoms	Exacerbations	Night symptoms	PEF or FEV$_1$% predicted	PEF variability
Step 1: mild, intermittent	<Once/week	Brief (few hours to few days)	<Twice/month	>80%	<20%
Step 2: mild, persistent	Once/week	May affect activity and sleep	>Twice/month	>80%	20–30%
Step 3: moderate, persistent	Daily	Affects activity and sleep	>Once/week	60–80%	>30%
Step 4: severe, persistent	Continuous	Frequent	Frequent	<60%	>30%

Table 2.1
Chronic asthma severity according to WHO–GINA guidelines

episodic asthma, fixed asthma, cough-variant asthma, asthma in remission and pre-asthma. Another component of severity that has been introduced is the concept of minimal asthma therapy needed to control asthma over a period of time, as used by the British Thoracic Society's asthma guidelines to classify the severity of asthma. In addition, terms such as corticosteroid-dependent or -resistant asthma are sometimes used to denote severe asthma. So far, indices derived from the inflammatory component of the disease have not been added to the assessment of severity. The overall severity of an asthmatic can be assessed from a combination of clinical, lung function, inflammatory and therapeutic factors, but the contribution of each of these factors in the assessment is difficult to determine.

A widely used classification of severity is the one used by the WHO–GINA guidelines (Table 2.1). Unfortunately, it remains unvalidated, in particular with respect to prognosis, to treatment outcomes and to quality-of-life measures. In addition, the link between lung function and the clinical features has not been established. The contribution of bronchial hyperresponsiveness and airway inflammation to the definition of severity is not known. For patients who experience frequent exacerbations but remain asymptomatic in between, the attack rate and the severity of each episode are useful indicators of severity. In fact, previous admission to hospital for treatment of an acute severe attack of asthma is a strong marker for subsequent risk of asthma death, and the risk increases with the number of previous admissions. In contrast to measurement of the chronic severity of asthma, the severity of an acute exacerbation can be measured more directly and accurately.

Investigations and laboratory assessment of asthma

Investigations and laboratory assessment are important adjuncts to history and examination for obtaining confirmation of variable airflow obstruction, assessing the severity of the asthma, evaluating the presence of allergic factors, determining structural changes to the airways and measuring the degree of airway inflammation. In addition, investigations and laboratory assessment are necessary to examine other potential concomitant or alternative diagnoses. This assessment is not necessary in the majority of patients, but is recommended for patients who present with features of severe asthma, often unresponsive to available asthma treatments. A comprehensive list of investigations is provided in Box 3.1. It is important to state that all these investigations and laboratory assessment are not usually necessary for most patients, apart from lung function tests; in the more severe patients, some of these tests may help in staging severity and in further management.

Lung function measurements to assess airflow limitation

Lung function test measurements are recommended for both the diagnosis and the assessment of the severity of asthma, and are of use for planning appropriate therapeutic measures. Patient symptoms and physical examination may not provide an accurate assessment of the severity of the asthma, and poor perception of asthma symptoms has been put forward as a potential reason for delays in obtaining treatment, which may contribute to increasing severity and deaths from asthma. With the development of portable instruments, lung function tests can be performed by the patient daily, and the diurnal variability of lung function measurements provides a good measure of asthma severity.

Although there is a wide range of different methods to assess the level of airflow limitation, only two methods have gained wide acceptance: forced

Box 3.1

Laboratory investigations and studies

1. Evaluation of severity of asthma:
   (a) spirometry (forced expiratory volume in one sec/forced vital capacity in one second; peak expiratory flow rate);
   (b) home recording of peak expiratory flow rate (PEFR).

2. Investigations supporting diagnosis of asthma, either inclusive or exclusive:
   (a) full blood count (eosinophilia);
   (b) chest radiograph;
   (c) examination for eosinophils in sputum (or induced sputum);
   (d) complete inspiratory and expiratory flow volume curve;
   (e) provocative challenge with occupational allergens;
   (f) measurement of bronchial responsiveness with methacholine, histamine or exercise.

3. Investigations of associated/risk factors:
   (a) examination of upper airways (nose, sinuses, pharynx);
   (b) evaluation of gastro-oesophageal reflux (pH studies, gatroscopic examination);
   (c) evaluation of the role of allergy with skin-prick tests, or with determination of specific IgE antibodies to common inhalant allergens or with determination of total IgE levels.

4. Inflammatory markers:
   (a) blood eosinophil counts;
   (b) serum eosinophil cationic protein (ECP);
   (c) eosinophils in induced sputum;
   (d) ECP levels in induced sputum;
   (e) exhaled nitric oxide level;
   (f) urinary leukotriene E_4 excretion.

expiratory volume in 1 second (FEV_1) with forced vital capacity (FVC), and the peak expiratory flow. These measurements are based on the concept of airflow limitation relating to the airway size and the elastic recoil properties of the lung parenchyma. Measurement of FEV_1 and FVC is made during a forced expiratory manoeuvre using a spirometer, and is effort-dependent (see below). Both FEV_1 and the FEV_1/FVC ratio are reduced during airflow obstruction (Figure 3.1).

Pulmonary function tests traditionally comprise measurements of lung volumes and of flow rates produced with maximum expiratory effort. Lung volumes are measured in the lung function laboratory, using either body plethysmographic or gas (helium) dilution methods. Using spirometric methods, the tidal volume, the vital capacity, the expiratory reserve volume and the inspiratory capacity of the lung can be determined. During an episode of airflow obstruction, or in chronic asthma, the lung volumes are

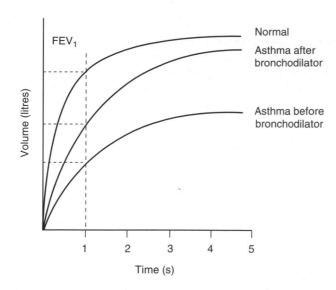

Figure 3.1
Forced expiratory volume with time curves in a normal subject and in an asthmatic with airflow obstruction. The FEV_1 is the volume measured in the first second. Note the bronchodilator response in the asthmatic following inhalation of a bronchodilator β-agonist.

usually increased, particularly the residual volume in relation to the vital capacity. Flow rates can be measured directly or by determining the volume expired over a period of time. The following indices can be obtained:

1. FVC, which is the total volume of air expired as rapidly as possible from one single expiration from total lung capacity.
2. FEV_1, which is the volume of air expired in 1 second from maximum inspiration, obtained from the same tracing as FVC. The ratio of FEV_1 to FVC is also used as an index of airflow limitation.
3. Peak expiratory flow rate (PEFR), which is the maximum flow rate that can be generated during a forced expiratory manoeuvre.
4. Maximum mid-expiratory flow rate (MMEF), which is the slope of the line between 25 and 75 per cent of the forced expiratory volume.

These tests are effort-dependent, and it is important to teach patients to be proficient in the technique of maximum exhalation. Use of an instrument that provides a flow-volume trace is useful in providing information on the adequacy of the inspiratory and expiratory manoeuvres, but this is not available on the portable peak flow meters.

FORCED EXPIRATORY VOLUME IN ONE SECOND (FEV₁)

It is useful to have a measurement of FEV_1 and FVC at the initial visit, since the FEV_1 is the single best reproducible measure of pulmonary function for assessing severity, and periodic measurements may be useful in following the patient's progress or response to treatment. A normal vital capacity with an impaired FEV_1 indicates airflow obstruction. In severe obstruction, both FEV_1 and FVC may be reduced, but the ratio of FEV_1 to FVC will be less than the normal ratio of 75 per cent (Figure 3.1). Use of the FEV_1 to FVC ratio will also provide evidence as to whether there is a restrictive defect, where the ratios are usually greater than 75 per cent. Measurement of mid-expiratory flow rate may provide evidence for small airways disease, although this measurement may be too sensitive to assess the severity of the obstruction.

PEAK EXPIRATORY FLOW RATE (PEFR)

Many general practices may not have access to a spirometer for measuring FEV_1, and the PEFR when performed well correlates well with FEV_1 and is more convenient to obtain. However, PEFR has limitations that need to be recognized. First, it is effort dependent, and proper training is essential to obtain the best and reproducible measurements from an individual patient. Second, the inter-individual variability of PEFR is wide and the predicted values available may not necessarily accurately reflect the 'normal' for a particular patient. It is more useful to establish a best PEFR for each patient during a period of monitoring when the patient is at his best ('best-ever PEFR'). Third, measurements of PEFR are likely to reflect mostly the calibre of the large airways rather than that of the small airways.

Against these limitations, the PEFR measurement has many benefits. Reliable, robust, portable and relatively inexpensive PEFR machines are now available and provide a reliable objective measurement of diurnal variation of airflow obstruction (Box 3.2). It is also important that the patient indicates

Box 3.2

Uses of peak expiratory flow rate (PEFR) machines

1. Regular monitoring for diagnosis or confirmation or exclusion of asthma.
2. Assess the severity of airflow obstruction, particularly when the 'usual normal' PEFR value is known for a particular patient.
3. Monitor diurnal variability of airflow obstruction.
4. Monitor response to therapy or overall success of treatment.
5. Monitor response to therapy during an acute attack of asthma treated at home.
6. Diagnose exercise-induced asthma by measuring PEFR before and after exercise.
7. Diagnose occupational asthma by measuring PEFR at and off the workplace.
8. Use to detect early signs of airflow obstruction, particularly in poor perceivers.
9. Use as part of an overall self-management plan with stepping up of treatments at specific values of PEFR measurements.

how soon prior to the measurement of PEFR he has taken bronchodilator therapy, since a post-bronchodilator PEFR measurement may mask the severity of asthma. PEF meter readings may change with extended use, and significant errors may occur in the reading range of many devices, with some over-reading in the middle flow range and under-reading at high flow ranges. Therefore, PEF devices must be checked regularly for accuracy and reproducibility of results. With attention to detail in performing PEFR and to accuracy, PEFR values can be useful in the follow-up of patients with asthma and in their response to therapy, by assessing variation in PEFR over days or weeks.

One indicator of asthma control is the degree of diurnal variation, which can be measured as the difference between the maximum and the minimum PEFR value from the daily morning and evening measurements expressed as a percentage of the mean PEFR (Figure 3.2a). An arbitrary limit of 20 per cent in diurnal variability is assumed as normal, while others suggest a greater than 12 per cent of the 95 per cent confidence interval of the mean percentage difference between the highest and lowest of four PEFR values measured in the morning and afternoon, before and after using a bronchodilator. A high variation above 20 per cent is usually taken to indicate poor asthma control. A simpler index is being advocated, which is the lowest PEFR, expressed as a percentage of the patient's known best PEFR. During an exacerbation, a linear fall in PEFR values over several days, with normal diurnal variability, is often observed. Therefore, poor asthma control and asthma exacerbations provide different patterns of PEFRs which can be distinguished.

In some patients, the measurements may be more sensitive than the development of symptoms, and therefore can be used to detect earlier the onset of an exacerbation of asthma in some patients (Figure 3.2b) so that preventive treatment can be instituted. Self-monitoring of PEFR may also be useful in relating worsening episodes of asthma to certain allergic or occupational exposures. The PEFR remains a very useful instrument for the assessment and diagnosis of occupational asthma.

BRONCHODILATOR RESPONSES TO PHARMACOLOGICAL AGENTS

Asthma is characterized by improvements in airflow obstruction following administration of β-agonists and corticosteroids. This can be demonstrated by an improvement in FEV_1 20–30 minutes after an inhaled short-acting $β_2$-agonist (200–400 μg of inhaled salbutamol), or after a 7- to 14-day course of inhaled or oral prednisolone (30–40 mg/day) (Figure 3.3). A 12 per cent or greater improvement in FEV_1 of at least 180 mL from baseline after an inhaled β-agonist is considered significant, but not necessarily indicative of asthma. Usually a greater than 15 per cent improvement is considered diagnostic of asthma. An increase of more than 20 per cent in FEV_1, and at least

Figure 3.2
(a) Variability in peak expiratory flow rates in an asthmatic subject, showing the typical worsening in the mornings. (b) Fall in peak expiratory flow rate during an exacerbation of asthma. Symptoms usually occur concomitantly or sometimes follow the onset of the fall in PEF. There is a gradual recovery over 7–10 days with treatment.

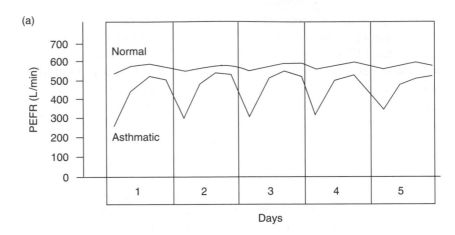

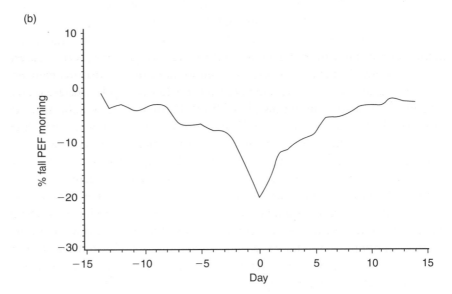

250 mL above baseline, after a course of prednisolone is taken as a positive response, supporting a diagnosis of asthma. Similar changes are expected with measurement of PEFR.

BRONCHIAL RESPONSIVENESS

The airways of patients with asthma demonstrate bronchial hyperresponsiveness, which is the increased bronchoconstrictor response to a variety of physical, chemical and pharmacologic stimuli, such as histamine, methacholine, exercise and cold air. Although a few other airway conditions demonstrate this feature, such as allergic rhinitis with no asthma symptoms, COPD,

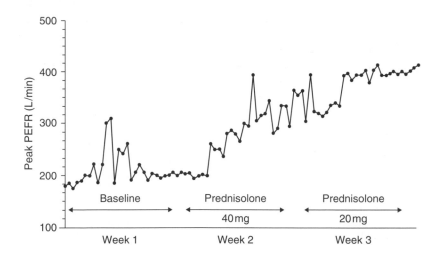

Figure 3.3
Improvement in peak expiratory flow rate (PEFR) during an exacerbation of asthma following treatment with a course of oral corticosteroids (prednisolone 40 mg/day for 1 week, followed by 20 mg/day for another week).

cystic fibrosis and sarcoidosis or even some asymptomatic people, it is most commonly observed in asthma, even in mild asthma patients with normal lung function. Changes in pulmonary function, usually FEV_1, are measured after inhaling each incremental dose of a bronchoconstrictor substance such as methacholine or histamine. Results are expressed as the cumulative dose (PD_{20}) or the concentration of bronchoconstrictor agent (PC_{20}) needed to cause a 20 per cent fall in FEV_1 (Figure 3.4). A PC_{20}-FEV_1 methacholine or histamine greater than 16 mg/mL is usually considered to be normal.

In children, exercise provocation is often preferred as a more natural stimulus and is usually better tolerated. Exercise may take the form of free running outside or up the stairs. Usually a small degree of bronchodilatation can be observed during the exercise period, and bronchoconstriction appears within seconds of stopping exercise (Figure 3.5). A standardized form of exercise is required to document the severity and evaluate the effects of therapy. The results of exercise provocation are expressed as maximal fall in FEV_1 after exercise. Isocapnic hyperventilation with dry air is sometimes used in some laboratories, obviating the need for exercise.

In most asthmatics, bronchial hyperresponsiveness is present. However, exposure to allergens or occupational agents can lead to an increase in bronchial hyperresponsiveness, and spontaneous worsening of asthma symptoms is also accompanied by such an increase. Some patients with a presumed diagnosis of asthma because of mild symptoms may have a normal bronchial responsiveness to methacholine or histamine, and up to 9 per cent of such subjects develop asthma within 10 years. On the other hand, 10 per cent of normal people demonstrate bronchial hyperresponsiveness, and nearly half of those develop asthma within 2 years of follow-up, indicating that bronchial hyperresponsiveness may be a risk factor for developing asthma.

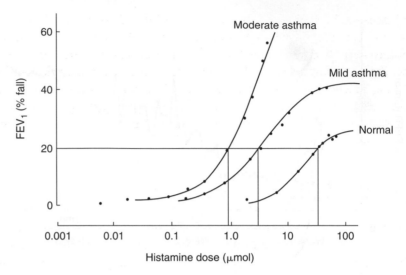

Figure 3.4
Fall in FEV_1 with incremental concentrations of inhaled histamine in two asthmatic patients and a normal volunteer, showing a shift of the concentration response to the left in the asthmatic subjects, indicating increased sensitivity. The PC_{20} is the concentration of histamine needed to cause a 20 per cent fall in FEV_1. Note also that the maximum response in terms of fall in FEV_1 is greater in the asthmatic compared to the normal subjects. In the moderate asthmatic, this 'plateau' response may not be achieved. (Adapted from Woolcock *et al.* (1984) *Am. Rev. Respir. Dis.* **130**, 71–5.)

Figure 3.5
Changes in peak expiratory flow rates (PEFR) in an asthmatic child during and following exercise.

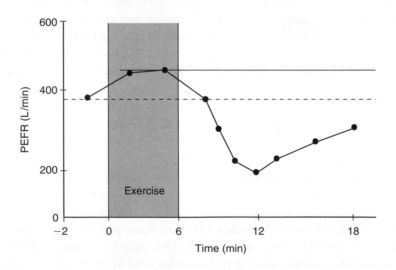

Clinically, the most common indication for measuring bronchial responsiveness is for providing support or for excluding a diagnosis of asthma in patients where the history is vague or atypical. It is not known whether monitoring of bronchial responsiveness may be an effective way of measuring asthma severity or of response to treatments. Treatment with inhaled corticosteroid therapy improves bronchial hyperresponsiveness but rarely normalizes bronchial responsiveness. Treatment aimed at reducing bronchial hyperresponsiveness, rather than just symptoms, may lead to a better control of asthma exacerbations and lung function, with a greater reduction in airway inflammation, which emphasizes the importance of measuring bronchial responsiveness to monitor therapeutic responses. However, the use of bronchial responsiveness as an adjunct to measuring response to treatment is not generally recommended at present.

Quality-of-life measures

In a chronic disease such as asthma, particularly those with persistent symptoms, health-related quality-of-life measures provide an indication of how the disease is affecting the patient. This measure includes a set of physical and psychological characteristics assessing the problems in the social context of a patient's lifestyle. It may be general or disease specific. General health measures are standardized and compare the burden of illness across different medical conditions. However, for a condition like asthma, these general health measures are not sensitive enough to small, but clinically important, changes produced by asthma. Disease-specific questionnaires for asthma are available, such as the Asthma Quality of Life Questionnaire (AQLQ), and are more sensitive to change, and a minimal increase or decrease in the score that has clinical relevance has been defined. Using this questionnaire, the quality-of-life scores were correlated with morning peak flow and with the severity of asthma, but there was no relationship to the level of physical activity. In patients with severe asthma, worse than expected quality-of-life scores may be obtained, which do not relate to the level of airflow obstruction as measured by FEV_1 or variation in peak flow. Some improvement in quality-of-life scores can be seen with treatment with bronchodilators or anti-inflammatory treatments. Therefore, quality-of-life scores provide measures that do not only reflect physiological disturbances, but the overall physical and psychological impacts on the patient of the chronic disease. These measurements are not currently used routinely in the clinical assessment of patients with asthma, but may become a useful parameter.

Assessment of risk factors

ALLERGENS AND ALLERGY

Exposure to allergens is a most important risk factor for developing allergic diseases and asthma, and for provoking an episode of asthma in those with allergies (see Chapter 4). Allergens sensitize atopic individuals by causing the development of specific T-cell clones and the production of specific IgE antibodies.

Once sensitized, an individual is then prone to developing allergic inflammation and asthma exacerbations on re-exposure to the allergen. There is a correlation between asthma prevalence and long-term allergen exposure, and improvements in asthma after cessation of exposure. An assessment of allergy remains an important part of the evaluation of the asthmatic patient.

The common aeroallergens important in causing asthma attacks can be categorized broadly into indoor allergens, such as house dust mite, animal allergens and fungi, and outdoor allergens, including pollen and fungi.

Allergens

House dust mites

House dust mites are present worldwide, and are a major cause of asthma. In addition to their potential allergenic effects, they have been identified as being cysteine protease enzymes and therefore, when deposited on the epithelial surface, may breakdown epithelial barriers to reach the submucosal surfaces where immunocompetent cells are present. A relationship between symptoms and mite allergen exposure has been described, and the degree of exposure to mite in the first year of life correlates with the subsequent development of asthma. House dust mites consist principally of *Dermatophagoides pteronyssinus* and their excreta. Mites feed on human and animal scales colonized by microfungi, yeasts and bacteria. They can be found on floors, but tend to bury deep in carpets, mattresses and soft furnishings. Temperatures between 22 and 26°C and a relative humidity of greater than 55 per cent are ideal conditions for growth for the house dust mite. *Dermatophagoides pteronyssinus* is the most dominant mite found in damp climates. *Blomia tropicalis* is more commonly found in tropical or subtropical countries such as Brazil. *Dermatophagoides farinae*, present in flour, survives better in drier climates. A concentration of mite allergen above 2 μg/g of dust is considered as a significant risk factor for the development of allergy.

Cat allergens

The principal cat allergen, *Fel d1*, is a potent sensitizer and is found in the cat pelt, produced by the sebaceous glands. Cat saliva is also another potent source. The allergen is carried in small respirable particles. Dust from houses with a cat contains 10–1500 μg of *Fel d1*.

Dog allergens

Up to 30 per cent of allergic persons have positive skin tests to dog extracts. A dog allergen has been purified from dog hair and dander. *Cad1* is present in large concentrations in saliva.

Fungi

Alternaria has been established as a risk factor of asthma in different populations and has been associated with the risk of asthma deaths. Indoor fungi include *Aspergillus, Alternaria, Cladosporium* and *Candida. Alternaria* and *Cladosporium* are also present outdoors.

Cockroaches and mice

In inner cities, particularly in lower socioeconomic dwellings, cockroaches are an important indoor allergen. A high proportion of asthma and rhinitis patients from inner city areas in major US cities have positive skin tests to cockroach extract. Similarly, there has been evidence of sensitization to urine proteins from mice in inner city dwellers.

Pollen

The concentration of pollen in air varies with location and atmospheric conditions. Usually tree pollen predominates in early spring, grass pollen in late spring and summer, and weed pollen during summer and autumn. Pollen allergens are carried in large particles, but smaller respirable particles of starch granules are released from pollen, particularly after rainfall. These have been implicated in asthma epidemics that may follow thunderstorms.

Diagnosis of allergy

The history should include the patient's lifestyle and occupational history, which influence exposure to particular allergens or chemicals, the timing of the exposure, and the relationship between exposure and the development of symptoms of asthma and/or ocular and nasal symptoms. The presence of pets at home and the state of the house (carpets, pillows, bedding) should be ascertained. Collection of house dust in order to measure house dust mite levels is currently a research exercise, but this is the only measure of the degree of exposure available for this common aeroallergen. The degree of exposure often relates to the degree of symptoms. The role of food allergy or food additives remains unclear, but should be investigated if there are any important reactions or asthma symptoms relating to certain foods.

Testing for allergies

Skin tests to common aeroallergens are the best test for the diagnosis of allergy, because of their simplicity, ease and rapidity of performance, and also because of their diagnostic sensitivity and specificity. The common aeroallergens usually tested are: house dust mite, grass pollen, tree pollen, cat, dog and aspergillus. Skin-prick tests, performed by pricking the skin of the patient through a drop of allergen extract, are reproducible and safe. A positive (histamine 10 mg/mL) and negative (diluent) control are also included when performing these tests. Positive tests are characterized by a wheal, usually greater than 2 mm in diameter, with a negative response to the diluent solution (Figure 3.6).

The most commonly used serological allergy tests are measurements of total and specific IgE antibodies to allergens relevant to the patient's symptoms.

Figure 3.6
Wheal and erythema formation in the forearm skin of an allergic asthmatic patient, following skin-prick tests with a series of aeroallergens such as house dust mite and grass pollen.

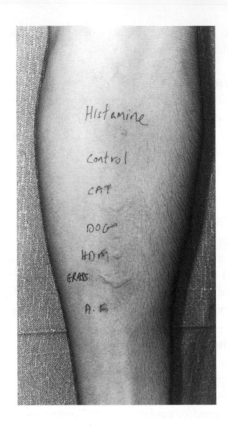

Allergen-specific IgE antibodies, usually measured by immunoassay (radioaller-gosorbent test, RAST) or by immunoenzyme assay (enzyme-linked immuno-sorbent assay, ELISA), are more expensive and yet not as sensitive as prick tests. *In vitro* measurement of total IgE is useful in that these levels are usually elevated in allergic subjects.

Allergen provocation tests

The relevance of particular allergens can only be determined by exposing the patient to aerosols of the aeroallergen in question in a provocation test. This can only be performed in specialized centres under close supervision. Usually, these challenges are performed for research purposes, such as for the investigation of the effects of potential new drugs for asthma, using the effects of allergen expo-sure as a reproducible controlled exacerbation of asthma. From the diagnostic point of view, inhalational challenges are often performed for the diagnosis of occupational asthma where the worker is exposed to the substances he encoun-ters at work (for example, small molecular weight sensitizers such as isocyanates or trimellitic anhydride). Often, exposures to allergen provoke an immediate bronchoconstrictor response (the early response) which usually disappears by 30–60 minutes, followed sometimes by a more persistent, sometimes severe,

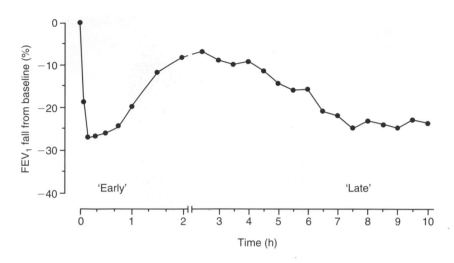

Figure 3.7
Changes in FEV_1 following inhalation of house dust mite allergen in a mild allergic asthmatic patient showing an immediate early bronchoconstrictor response followed by a late response.

episode of bronchoconstriction (late-phase response) 8–12 hours later (Figure 3.7). Allergen provocation tests can therefore be dangerous and should only be performed under the strictest supervision.

RADIOLOGICAL ASSESSMENT

Radiological assessment of the nose and sinuses may be necessary to ascertain the degree of rhinitis and sinusitis, using sinus CT scans. The airways and lungs may also be visualized by using high-resolution CT scans. In chronic asthma, the intrapulmonary airways may show dilatation with a thickened airway wall (Figure 3.8), but the pathological correlates of these radiological changes are not known and the contribution of these changes to the severity of asthma is unclear. This test can be used to exclude or confirm the diagnosis of frank bronchiectasis. Other changes, rarely observed, include mucus plugging. However, more commonly, air trapping can be seen, particularly when scans taken at inspiration and at expiration are compared, and the degree of air trapping relates to the severity of airflow obstruction. Localized areas of emphysema are also described. The clinical value of the chest CT scan in asthma lies in differentiating asthma from COPD, and in excluding the diagnosis of frank bronchiectasis.

Airway inflammation

Airway inflammation is an important characteristic feature of asthma, and its investigation has led to a better understanding of the pathogenesis of asthma, and to improved treatment strategies. The assessment of airway inflammation at the clinical level has been made possible by the development of repeatable

Figure 3.8
High-resolution computed tomogram of an asthma patient, showing the presence of thickened and dilated intrapulmonary airways.

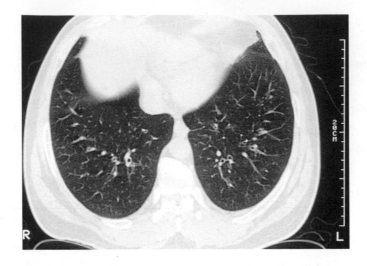

non-invasive techniques, such as induced sputum and exhaled nitric oxide. Although these techniques are not currently being used routinely to assess airway inflammation, several studies suggest that they may play a role in diagnosis, in the assessment of severity of asthma and in measuring therapeutic responses to drugs.

The use of fibreoptic bronchoscopy for retrieving mucosal biopsies from the large airways and for obtaining bronchoalveolar cells from the distal airways has provided important findings regarding the constituents of the cellular inflammatory process. The characteristic pathological picture includes a variable patchy loss of the surface epithelium, a thickening of the epithelial reticular basement membrane and an increased cellular infiltrate in the mucosa, represented by activated eosinophils and also by mast cells and T cells. However, fibreoptic bronchoscopy remains a research technique used in a few research centres, and cannot presently be recommended as a routine test for measuring airway inflammation.

INDUCED SPUTUM

Induction of sputum by inhalation of hypertonic saline has proved to be a reliable and reproducible method for analysing inflammatory cells from the major airways of patients. The method of sputum induction is generally safe, although patients should be monitored with FEV_1 measurements to detect any important bronchospasm, which can be treated promptly with bronchodilators. The collected expectorate represents a mixture of saliva, mucus and airway liquids, and the cells can either be examined from selected macroscopic mucus plugs or from the whole expectorate, after they have been dispersed with dithiothreitol. A differential cell count can be performed on cytospin preparations of the cell suspension. The fluid phase of the expectorate can be

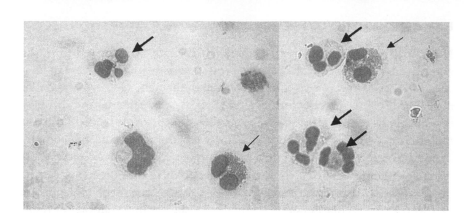

Figure 3.9
Cells obtained from induced sputum of a patient with asthma, showing eosinophils (thin arrows) and neutrophils (thick arrows).

assayed for various mediators, such as eosinophil-derived proteins (e.g. eosinophil cationic protein or eosinophil peroxidase) or neutrophil-derived proteins (such as neutrophil myeloperoxidase or elastase).

Cell counts of induced sputum from normal individuals show predominance of macrophages and neutrophils, with only the occasional eosinophil, lymphocyte and epithelial cells. In adults and children with asthma, there is an increase in the proportion and numbers of eosinophils, metachromatic cells and sometimes neutrophils (Figure 3.9), while, in the fluid phase, increased concentrations of eosinophilic proteins, such as eosinophil cationic protein (ECP) and eosinophil peroxidase, in addition to markers of increased microvascular permeability such as albumin and fibrinogen, have been measured. The degree of sputum eosinophilia and amount of eosinophilic products are also higher in symptomatic, compared to asymptomatic, asthmatics. The degree of sputum eosinophilia and levels of sputum ECP are increased during experimental induction of asthma worsening, either by withdrawal of inhaled corticosteroid treatment or through exposure of allergic asthmatics to allergens, or during spontaneous exacerbations of asthma. Thus, sputum eosinophilia may reflect disease activity, and may contribute to the assessment of severity. In addition, sputum eosinophilia is usually associated with a good clinical response to corticosteroids, while its absence indicates a poor response. In patients with chronic severe asthma and during acute exacerbations of asthma, the sputum may also show increased levels of neutrophils, which may be another marker of disease activity.

Therefore, serial measurements of sputum eosinophilia may provide an index of activity of the disease, providing an index of the therapeutic response to asthma treatments. By contrast, blood eosinophils and serum ECP levels are insensitive measurements of eosinophilic airway inflammation. Measurements of sputum eosinophilia holds promise, and it is not clear whether targeting treatments to suppress sputum eosinophilia may lead to better outcomes when compared to just controlling symptoms.

EXHALED NITRIC OXIDE

Nitric oxide is a gas that is present in exhaled breath. It is derived from the amino acid, L-arginine, by the action of nitric oxide synthases (NOS) in lung cells, such as epithelial cells and vascular endothelium. One type of NOS, inducible NOS, is increased in the airways of asthma patients, and this may form the basis of the increased levels of exhaled nitric oxide (eNO) found in their breath. Measuring eNO is very attractive because it can be done rapidly by most patients, by exhaling into a chemiluminescence analyser, and the test result is obtained immediately. As such, serial eNO measurements can be obtained easily, and very frequently, in the same patient. eNO levels are increased in several diseases other than asthma, such as upper and lower respiratory tract infections, pulmonary tuberculosis, bronchiectasis, and in non-asthmatic atopic patients. In cross-sectional studies of patients with asthma not receiving treatment with inhaled corticosteroids, eNO correlated with airway hyperresponsiveness and sputum eosinophil counts; however, this was not seen in patients treated with corticosteroids. eNO levels have been correlated with asthma symptoms over the past 2 weeks, a dyspnoea score, daily use of rescue medication and reversibility of airflow obstruction. There have been no longitudinal studies to assess its use as a daily marker of asthma severity or control, and it is too early to recommend it.

Mechanisms of asthma: risk factors and pathophysiology

Over the past 30 years, the central role that airway inflammation plays in the development of bronchial hyperresponsiveness and bronchial obstruction in asthma has been recognized. Continuing basic research in asthma in recent years has elucidated the basic steps that lead to the chronic inflammatory processes found in asthma and how these inflammatory processes can induce the physiological abnormalities that characterize asthma. The research approaches to asthma, a problem with such potentially diverse aetiologies, are necessarily multidisciplinary and often involve epidemiology, genetics, biochemistry, immunology, cell and molecular biology, pathology and physiology. Recent advances in the immunology of the T cell has allowed researchers to focus on the early events surrounding the acquisition of the allergic or asthmatic phenotype, an understanding of which may lead to prevention, or possibly cure, of allergies and asthma. Many potential new targets for the treatment of asthma have been identified, and one of the main aims of asthma research is to develop newer, more effective therapies. The questions that have been formulated in trying to understand the mechanisms of asthma are:

1. What are the risk factors for developing asthma? Identification of such risk factors may lead to identification of the early abnormalities.
2. Once asthma is established, what are the processes that lead to the chronic inflammatory changes, including chronic airway remodelling?
3. What is the underlying pathophysiology of airway wall narrowing and of bronchial hyperresponsiveness?

Risk factors for asthma

The predisposing factors for development of asthma may be divided into genetic or environmental factors such as exposure to sensitizing aeroallergens or environmental pollutants (Figure 4.1). Consistent with asthma being influenced by genetic factors are data from studies of twins, showing that the susceptibility to asthma accounted for by genetic influences is of the

Figure 4.1
Influence of genetic
and environmental
factors on airway
inflammation, bronchial
hyperresponsiveness
and bronchoconstriction.

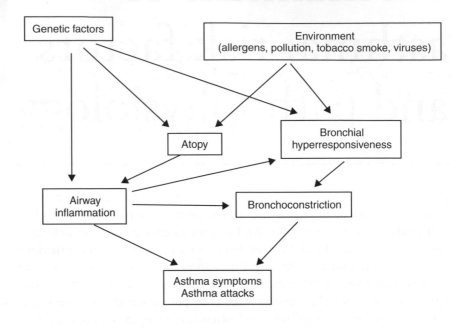

order of 0.4–0.8. This allows for an important contribution of environmental factors. Genes linked to asthma may be identified either by a process known as positional cloning or by examining candidate genes. Using family data, linkage analysis has been used to determine the location of susceptibility genes. Efforts are being made to make a systematic identification of these genes throughout the genome, but this has shown the complexity of genetic susceptibility interacting with several environmental factors, which could explain the variable phenotypic features of asthma across the population. Asthma is a polygenic disease that represents a complex interaction between predisposing factors that increase the susceptibility and causal factors that induce an asthma response. For example, some of the genetic factors underlying the atopic state have been identified, and once the airways have been sensitized, exposure to causal factors, such as inhaled allergens, can induce an episode of bronchoconstriction. In addition, genetic susceptibility to bronchial hyperresponsiveness may increase the effect of other causal factors, such as exposure to cigarette smoke, air pollution and upper respiratory tract viral infections (Figure 4.1).

ATOPY AND GENETIC PREDISPOSITION

The majority of children and adults with asthma are atopic, as defined by having either positive skin-prick tests to various common inhalant allergens or raised amounts of circulating IgE levels. A significant number do not have identifiable atopy. Epidemiological studies show that the prevalence of asthma increases with increasing levels of IgE, and those with low serum IgE levels have low prevalence of asthma. However, asthma is associated in only a proportion of atopic individuals, since the prevalence of atopy in the population is of the order of 30–50 per cent while that of asthma is lower. This suggests that there may be local factors (e.g. in the airways) that interact with circulating levels of IgE to cause asthma. Closely associated with raised serum IgE levels are bronchial hyperresponsiveness and asthma. Using the criteria that both high serum IgE and specific serum IgE define atopy, one study found that in both nuclear and extended families, the distribution of atopic subjects was consistent with an autosomal dominant inheritance, identified at a gene located on chromosome 11. This gene could only exert its effect if inherited from the mother, an effect called genomic imprinting.

Linkage studies indicate that several chromosomal regions are likely to contain genes for allergy or asthma, including chromosomes 5q, 6p, 11q, 12q, 13q and 16q. For example, the cytokine gene cluster on 5q 23–31 contains numerous candidate genes for atopy, including those for IL-4 and IL-13, which are both key components necessary for the induction of IgE production. The location of the gene for the β-subunit of the high-affinity IgE receptor, FcϵRIβ is on chromosome 11q, while the gene for inteferon-γ (IFNγ), which has multiple roles in the immune response, is on chromosome 12q. An association of polymorphisms of the promoter region of the IL-4R gene on chromosome 16p with atopy and atopic asthma has been described. Therefore, a more complex picture of the hereditary mechanisms of asthma is emerging from statistical analysis of large samples of nuclear families, and, using linkage studies, from the large number of possible loci linked to asthma that spread across the genome. These observations indicate the complex interactions between different sets of genetic variants. Various factors known to be involved in the regulation of IgE and its effects are likely to be important in underlying atopy and asthma.

ALLERGEN EXPOSURE

Allergen exposure has been proposed as an important determinant of the risk of developing allergy and asthma. The increase in the prevalence of asthma has been paralleled by an increase in allergic rhinitis, indicating that the common denominator of these allergic diseases is allergic sensitization. Sensitization by exposure to usually indoor allergens, such as pollen, pets and house dust mite, and early feeding with foreign proteins, has been strongly associated with the development of asthma. Exclusive breast-feeding until at least 4 months of age significantly reduces the risk of childhood asthma assessed at age the age of 6, an effect that may result from exclusion of potentially allergenic components in early life. The degree of exposure to house dust mite during the first 2 years of life has been associated with the likelihood of developing asthma by the age of 11 years. The level of exposure can also be a factor, since changes in lifestyle, particularly living in well-insulated and enclosed spaces, as in Western societies, have led to increased exposure to house dust mite allergens. Levels of exposure may not be the only factor underlying the increased prevalence of allergic sensitization, since other studies have not shown a correlation between allergen exposure and the prevalence of asthma. In large prospective studies, the development of childhood asthma was not related to cat or mite allergen exposure in the first years of life, but sensitization to mite and cat allergens was associated with indoor allergen exposure. On the other hand, allergic sensitization to indoor allergens is associated with the prevalence of bronchial hyperresponsiveness and asthma. Thus, the link between allergen exposure, development of sensitization and acquisition of asthma needs to be looked at more carefully. Other consequences of the Western style of living that may have a bearing on the prevalence of asthma include dietary factors such as high salt intake, obesity and less exercise.

RESPIRATORY INFECTIONS

Viral respiratory infections, including rhinoviruses, respiratory syncytial virus (RSV), adenovirus, parainfluenza and influenza viruses, can provoke episodes of wheezing, that can evolve into severe attacks of asthma, particularly in children less than 3 years of age. More than 20 per cent of infants respond with a recurring wheeze that resolves in later childhood. These infants have reduced lung function before the onset of viral infection, have normal immune responses to viruses and do not have risk factors for asthma such as bronchial hyperresponsiveness or increased IgE levels. A second group of about 10 per cent of wheezy infants, also wheeze with virus infections but have some, or all, risk factors for asthma and have recurrent wheeze in later childhood. Lower respiratory tract infections associated with viral infections go on to develop recurrent episodes of airway obstruction and asthma during later childhood. The risk of continued wheezing is greater in infants hospitalized with proven bronchiolitis due to RSV. RSV infections may be a causative factor in the development of asthma in some children; it is associated with IgE production, airway inflammation and increased airways responsiveness. Infants who respond to RSV infection with lower respiratory tract illness and wheeze are likely to have an atopic background and to have asthma by 6 years of age.

TOBACCO SMOKE

Passive smoking is a well-identified risk factor for the development of allergic disease, particularly in early childhood, although maternal smoking may have the greatest effect. In addition, asthmatic children of smoking mothers have more severe asthma than those whose mothers are non-smokers. Exposure to cigarette smoke is associated with increased frequency and severity of exacerbations of asthma, and the development of asthma in predisposed infants and young children. The effects of cigarette smoke may also occur as early as in the intrauterine period.

RESPIRATORY IRRITANTS OR POLLUTANTS

A study in the former East and West Germany, performed soon after the German reunification, did not relate air pollution to an increased prevalence of allergies or asthma: the prevalence of allergic asthma was lower in East Germany, where exposure to pollution was the highest. However, episodes of high pollution have been related to an increase in asthma attacks, and pollution may augment airway responses induced by allergens. There are strong associations between ambient concentrations of inhalable particulates (diameter 10 μm, PM_{10}) and emergency room visits, admission to hospital and doctor visits for asthma. Increases in ozone concentrations in ambient air have also been associated with more emergency room visits and admissions to hospital for asthma. Ozone itself can induce airway inflammation, usually neutrophilic, although an increase in mucosal eosinophils can also be observed in atopic asthmatics. In atopic individuals, exposure to ozone increases the inflammation and the bronchial responsiveness induced by a subsequent exposure to allergen. Air pollutants have an adjuvant effect in the formation of IgE antibodies and cytokines. Diesel exhaust particles enhance IgE production by tonsillar B cells in the presence of factors needed for IgE synthesis, such as interleukin-4 and CD40 monoclonal antibody, and increase the expression of T-helper 2 (Th2) cytokines (IL-4, IL-5, IL-6, IL-10 and IL-13), but inhibit the T-helper 1 (Th1) cytokine, IFNγ, in nasal tissues. In animal experiments, intratracheal immunization with antigen in the presence of exhaust particles enhanced local IgE antibody production and also increased infiltration of eosinophils and the production of Th2 cytokines locally in the lungs, compared with either antigen or diesel exhaust particles alone.

CHRONIC STRESS

Stress as caused by parenting difficulties, such as parental anxiety and poor coping, may predict the onset of asthma by the age of 3 years in children at risk. High levels of stress also predict higher overall asthma morbidity in children, and has been associated with a higher frequency of upper respiratory tract infections, which are a known cause of asthma exacerbations. Severe negative life events increase the likelihood of new asthma exacerbations. Adverse psychosocial factors, including domestic and financial stresses, have been recognized as important risks associated with near-fatal asthma and asthma deaths. The mechanisms are not clearly understood.

Chronic airways inflammation of asthma: role of T-helper 2 cells and cytokines

Much of the understanding of the immunology of asthma has been derived from a close examination of the chronic inflammatory process of asthma, which is characterized by infiltration of the airway wall by diverse effector cells, including T lymphocytes, eosinophils, monocytes/macrophages and mast cells, and occasionally, neutrophils (Figure 4.2a). In addition, during exacerbations, an acute inflammatory process of asthma is often superimposed on the chronic inflammatory process, with extensive plasma extravasation and oedema, infiltration of the airway mucosa with eosinophils and neutrophils, and desquamation of the airway wall epithelium (Figure 4.2b). The mobilization, activation and trafficking of these effector cells to the airway are controlled by a complex cytokine milieu derived from activated $CD4^+$ T-helper (Th) cells and also from other resident airway cells, including airway smooth muscle and epithelial cells. Th cells of the type 2 variety secrete a Th2 profile of cytokines after cognate stimulation of the naïve T cell by antigen-presenting cells, such as the dendritic cell and the alveolar macrophage (Figure 4.3). The Th2 cytokine repertoire includes IL-4, IL-5, IL-9, IL-10 and IL-13. These cytokines promote various elements of allergic inflammation, including propagation of the Th2 phenotype, isotype-switching from IgG_1 to IgE synthesis, eosinophil mobilization, maturation and activation,

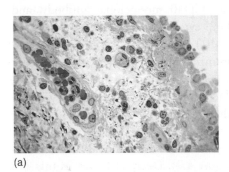

(a)

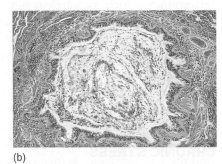

(b)

Figure 4.2
(a) Section from a fibreoptic bronchoscopic biopsy taken from a patient with symptomatic asthma, showing the presence of inflammatory cells within the airway mucosa, together with a desquamated epithelium. (b) Section from an airway taken from a patient who died during a severe attack of asthma, showing acute inflammatory changes in the airway wall with engorgement of the blood vessels, airway oedema, prominent airway smooth muscle bundles, and infiltration with inflammatory cells. The airway lumen is completely occluded by a mucus plug containing inflammatory cells and desquamated epithelium.

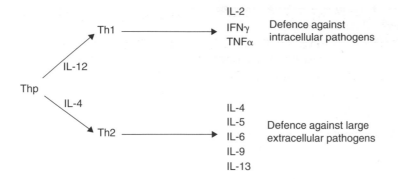

Figure 4.3
Differentiation of a T-helper progenitor (Thp) cell into either a T-helper 1 (Th1) or T-helper 2 (Th2) lineage, and the cytokines they express.

and mast cell activation. Additionally, the airway wall undergoes variable chronic changes, referred to as remodelling.

T-HELPER CELL IMBALANCE: Th2 POLARIZATION

T-cell profiles in the newborn demonstrate a bias towards Th2 cells, suggesting that prenatal influences are involved in T-cell priming. Th1 cells form a natural counterbalance to Th2 cells and are induced on exposure to foreign agents, including protozoa, bacteria and viral particles. Th1 responses are characterized by the induction of cell-mediated immune responses and the synthesis of IgG_{2a}, while Th2 responses are of humoral type, inciting the production of IgE and IgG_1. Th1 responses inhibit Th2 responses through the production of cytokines, including IL-12 and IFNγ. Delayed postnatal maturation of the cellular immune function may be a key determinant of genetic predisposition to atopic disease. This is based on the observation that neonates with a positive atopic family history and a greater risk of developing atopic disease have diminished capacity to secrete Th1 cytokines such as IFNγ and an increased capacity to produce Th2 cytokines, compared to neonates with a negative family history. There is preferential skewing to expansion of the $CD4^+$ Th2 lymphocyte subset in allergic processes, which may be the crucial forerunner to development of allergic disease. During the course of maturation of the normal infant, however, increased Th1 expression occurs, and the Th2 imbalance is overcome (Figure 4.4). Delay or failure of this Th1 response results in Th2 persistence and atopy or atopic disease, with a Th2 cytokine profile of IL-4, IL-5 and IL-13.

On the other hand, exposure to allergen during a particular sensitization window during infancy may predispose towards the development of long-term Th2-skewed allergen-specific immunological memory. Tolerance to repeated low-level inhaled aeroallergens may involve the activation of additional subsets of T cells that act as suppressor cells. These cells may cause Th2/Th1 switch or suppress both Th1 and Th2 responses. The failure of this process to occur naturally in atopic individuals is likely to result from a combination of allergic

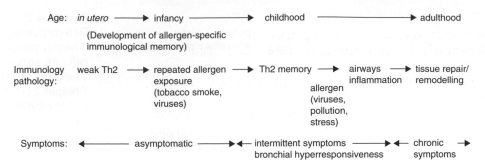

Figure 4.4
The immunological changes underlying allergy and asthma in relation to the natural history of asthma.

genetic predisposition and persistent stimulation by aeroallergens at a critical phase of immune maturation. Figure 4.4 depicts the immunological changes that may occur with the development of allergy and asthma.

In addition, certain childhood infections may protect against the development of atopy. An inverse relationship has been found between the development of measles infection in childhood and subsequent sensitization to house dust mite, while atopy in 12-year-old Japanese children is inversely related to delayed hypersensitivity to tuberculin. Infections may upregulate the production of Th1 cytokines to counterbalance any Th2 responses associated with allergic asthma. The impact of antibiotic use, changes in infections and vaccination practices may have influenced the prevalence of allergic asthma. Respiratory allergy is less frequent in those heavily exposed to oro-faecal and food-borne microbes. Thus, improved hygiene ('hygiene hypothesis') and a Westernized or semi-sterile diet may facilitate atopy by influencing exposure to commensals and pathogens that stimulate immune cell populations such as gut-associated lymphoid tissue. It has been proposed that children who are no longer exposed to commensals and pathogens become prone to the development of allergy and asthma. Early environmental exposure may be a determinant of the development of adult atopy, with influences that stimulate either a Th1 or Th2 response.

ROLE OF CYTOKINES

Cytokines are extracellular signalling proteins and are produced by different cell types involved in cell-to-cell interactions, having an effect on closely adjacent cells. Cytokines play an integral role in the coordination and persistence of the chronic allergic inflammatory process in asthma. They act on target cells to cause a wide array of cellular functions, including activation, proliferation, chemotaxis, immunomodulation, release of other cytokines or mediators, growth and cell differentiation, and apoptosis. Classification of cytokines

Box 4.1
Cytokines in asthma

1. Lymphokines: IL-2, IL-3, IL-4, IL-5, IL-13, IL-15, IL-16, IL-17.
2. Pro-inflammatory cytokines: IL-1, TNF, IL-6, IL-11, GM-CSF, SCF.
3. Anti-inflammatory cytokines: IL-10, IL-1ra, IFNγ, IL-12, 1L-18.
4. Chemotactic cytokines (chemokines):
   (a) eosinophils: CC chemokines (eotaxin, RANTES, MCP-4), GM-CSF;
   (b) monocytes/macrophages: MCP-1, MIP-1α, RANTES;
   (c) T cells: IL-16 (CD4$^+$), MIP-1α (CD8$^+$), STCP-1 (Th2), RANTES (memory), MCP-1, -3 and -4.
5. Growth factors: PDGF, TGFβ, FGF, EGF, IGF.

with regard to airways disease is best considered functionally, such as pro-inflammatory cytokines, T-cell derived cytokines, chemoattractant cytokines (chemokines) for eosinophils, neutrophils, monocytes/macrophages and T cells, anti-inflammatory cytokines and growth factors (Box 4.1).

Lymphokines

Originally, lymphokines which are soluble factors generated by activated lymphocytes, particularly CD4$^+$ T cells, in response to specific or polyclonal antigen were described, and formed the most important class of cytokines involved in immunological mechanisms. Particular subsets of CD4$^+$ T cells may be induced preferentially, secreting defined patterns of cytokines, resulting in initiation and propagation of distinct immune effector mechanisms. Studies in mouse CD4$^+$ T-cell clones, later in human CD4$^+$ T cells, have revealed two basic functional polarized subsets termed T-helper (Th) 1 and 2. Th1 T cells are characterized by predominant secretion of interleukin-2 (IL-2), IFN and tumour necrosis factor (TNF), triggering both cell-mediated immunity and production of opsonizing antibodies, while Th2 cells secrete predominantly IL-4, IL-5, IL-10 and IL-13, responsible for IgE and IgG$_4$ antibody production, and activation of mast cells and eosinophils. A third subset of Th cells, Thp (progenitor) cells, shows a composite profile, producing both Th1- and Th2-associated cytokines. In asthma, there is a predominance of expression of Th2-derived cytokines, such as IL-4, IL-5 and IL-13, leading to the hypothesis that asthma may result from an imbalance of Th2-derived cytokines (see above). In addition to CD4$^+$ T cells, CD8$^+$ T cells also have a similar dichotomy of expression of lymphokines.

Chemokines

Chemokines are chemotactic cytokines of 8–10 kDa involved in attracting leucocytes into tissues. Since the first chemokine, IL-8, was described in 1987, over 50 other chemokines have been recognized, encompassing four different structural families and interacting with at least 17 different receptors. The major families are CC chemokines (β-chemokines), in which two cysteine residues are adjacent to each other, and CXC chemokines (α-chemokines), in which these residues are separated by a non-conserved amino acid. The CC chemokines are involved in chemoattraction of eosinophils, monocytes and T lymphocytes, and are therefore of greatest relevance to asthma. Since the inflammatory pathology of asthma involves neutrophils, macrophages, T cells and occasionally eosinophils, chemokines that are involved in the chemoattraction of these cells are of interest. Of the CC chemokines, RANTES, macrophage inflammatory protein (MIP)-1α, monocyte chemoattractant protein (MCP)-1, MCP-3, MCP-4 and eotaxin may be involved. Eotaxin acting through the CCR3 receptor is a selective chemoattractant for eosinophils, while RANTES has a range of activities on memory T cells, basophils and eosinophils, acting through CCR1, CCR3 and CCR5 receptors. MCP-3 and -4 may recruit eosinophils and mononuclear cells, while MCP-1 can recruit monocytes, lymphocytes and basophils, and can activate mast cells and basophils.

Pro-inflammatory cytokines

In this group, the cytokines IL-1, TNF, IL-6 and granulocyte/macrophage colony stimulating factor (GM-CSF) may be included. IL-1 can be produced by a variety of cells, including monocytes/macrophages, fibroblasts, T cells, neutrophils and airway epithelial cells, although the major source is the monocyte/macrophage. IL-1, like TNF and IL-6, is an endogenous pyrogen. It partly causes leucocytosis by release of neutrophils from the bone marrow and induces the production of other cytokines, including IL-6, IL-8, RANTES, GM-CSF and TNF, from a variety of cells. It induces the expression of the adhesion molecules, intercellular adhesion molecule (ICAM)-1 and vascular cell adhesion molecule (VCAM)-1, on endothelial cells, which may lead to the increased adhesion of neutrophils and eosinophils to the vascular endothelium and respiratory epithelium. Many of the effects of IL-1β are similar to those of TNFα, which can stimulate airway epithelial cells to produce cytokines, including RANTES, IL-8 and GM-CSF. Both TNFα and IL-1β induce fibroblasts to proliferate, and IL-1β increases the synthesis of fibronectin and collagen.

GM-CSF is involved in priming inflammatory cells such as neutrophils and eosinophils, and can prolong the survival of eosinophils in culture. It induces the synthesis and release of a number of cytokines, such as IL-1 and TNFα, from monocytes.

Growth factors

Growth factors such as platelet-derived growth factor (PDGF), transforming growth factor (TGF)β and epidermal growth factor (EGF) influence the proliferation of many structural cells, such as fibroblasts and airway smooth muscle cells, and the turnover of matrix proteins. They may be involved in airway repair and remodelling processes.

EXPRESSION OF CYTOKINES IN ASTHMA

By using *in situ* hybridization technique to localize the expression of cellular messenger RNA, increased proportions of cells in bronchial biopsies and in bronchoalveolar lavage cells from patients with atopic asthma express genes for IL-3, IL-4, IL-5, IL-13 and GM-CSF when compared to those of non-atopic control subjects. In atopic asthmatics exposed to allergen, there is an increase in gene expression for these Th2 cytokines, but not for IFNγ, a Th1 cytokine, in bronchial biopsies and bronchoalveolar lavage cells. Lung T cells are activated and express and release high levels of Th2-type cytokines. The main cells expressing these cytokines are CD4$^+$ T cells, but mast cells also express IL-3, IL-4, IL-5, IL-6 and TNFα, and eosinophils, IL-5 and GM-CSF. Alveolar macrophages from patients with asthma also release more pro-inflammatory cytokines, IL-1β, TNFα, GM-CSF and MIP-1α when compared to those from normal subjects. The airway epithelium, which has for a while been considered to be functionally only a layer of cells providing a physical protective barrier, is metabolically active in expressing many proteins, particularly cytokines. In asthma, the airway epithelium overexpresses RANTES, eotaxin, IL-8 and GM-CSF. Therefore, although an excess of Th2 cytokines expressed in CD4$^+$ T cells is a most important abnormality in asthma, other cytokines are also overexpressed. How these cytokines are produced and act to increase cellular communications is shown in Figure 4.5.

ANTIGEN PRESENTATION AND RELEASE OF CYTOKINES

What are the primary signals that activate Th2 cells? These are related to the presentation of a restricted panel of antigens in the presence of appropriate cytokines. Allergens are taken up and processed by specialized cells within the mucosa, such as dendritic cells (antigen-presenting cells), followed by presentation of peptide fragments to naïve T cells. The activation of naïve T cells occurs, first via the CD4$^+$ T-cell receptor through the antigen-presenting cell (APC)-bound antigen to MHC II complex, and secondly, via the co-stimulatory pathway linked by the B7 family and T-cell-bound CD28. One ligand that binds to CD28, termed B7.2, induces T-cell activation and Th2 cell proliferation (Figure 4.6).

Cytokines play an important role in antigen presentation. Airway macrophages are usually poor at antigen presentation and suppress T-cell proliferative responses (possibly via release of cytokines such as IL-1 receptor

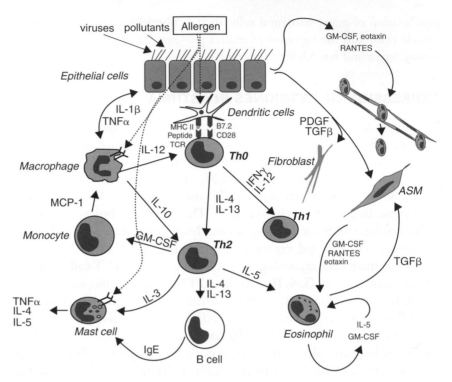

Figure 4.5
Potential cellular and cytokine interactions that may occur in asthma. Such interactions may be driven principally by allergens, with contributions from viruses and pollutants. The inflammation may be orchestrated by T-helper type 2 cells (Th2) which secrete cytokines such as IL-4 and IL-5, causing B cells to produce IgE and increasing eosinophil maturation and activation, respectively. Other cells, such as macrophages and mast cells, may contribute to this complex cellular interaction. The epithelium is likely to be another orchestrator of the inflammation. ASM, airway smooth muscle.

antagonist), but in asthma there is reduced suppression after exposure to allergen. Both GM-CSF and IFNγ increase the ability of macrophages to present allergen and express HLA-DR. IL-1 is important in activating T lymphocytes and is an important co-stimulator of the expansion of Th2 cells after antigen presentation. On exposure to inhaled allergens, airway mast cells and macrophages may become activated through the cross-linking of two high-affinity IgE receptors (FcεRI) on the surface of these cells by allergen, leading to the release of cytokines, such as IL-1, TNFα and IL-6. These cytokines may then act on epithelial cells to cause release of further cytokines, including GM-CSF, IL-8 and RANTES, which then leads to influx of secondary cells, such as eosinophils, which themselves may release multiple cytokines.

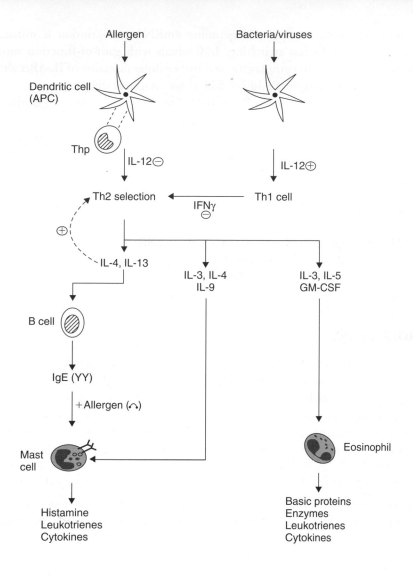

Figure 4.6
Effects of T-helper type 2 (Th2) clonal selection leading to production of IgE and mast cell degranulation, and to eosinophil recruitment and activation. Asthma and allergy may be considered as a disease with a Th2 overbalance. APC: antigen-presenting cell.

THE IMMUNOGLOBULIN E RESPONSE AND MAST CELLS

The cytokine IL-4, together with IL-13, is the most important cytokine involved in mediating IgE synthesis through isotype switching by B cells (Figures 4.5 and 4.6). IL-4 also activates B cells by increasing the expression of class II MHC molecules and of the low-affinity IgE (FcεRII) receptors. IL-4 also drives the differentiation of CD4$^+$ Th precursors into Th2-like cells. CD40 antigen is expressed on B cells after antigen recognition, and engagement with its ligand promotes IgE class switching and B-cell growth. IL-4 and IL-13 share the α chain of the IL-4 receptor (IL-4Rα). On engagement of the ligand with IL-4Rα, signal transducer and activator of transcription 6 (STAT 6) translocates to the nucleus and germline ϵmRNA transcription is initiated, together with IgE class switching. Individuals with gain-of-function mutations in both the extracytoplasmic and intracellular domains of IL-4Rα show an enhanced IgE response and predisposition to atopic disease.

IgE produced in asthmatic airways binds to FcϵRI receptors ('high affinity' IgE receptors) on mast cells and basophils, priming them for activation by antigen. Cross-linking of FcϵRI receptors upregulates their own expression and leads to mast cell degranulation, with the release of mediators such as histamine and cysteinyl-leukotrienes. The low-affinity IgE receptor, FcϵRII, or CD23, is present on B cells and many inflammatory cells, including macrophages and eosinophils, and seems to serve principally as a negative regulator of IgE synthesis.

The maturation and expansion of mast cells from bone marrow cells involves growth factors and cytokines, such as stem cell factor (SCF) and IL-3, derived from structural cells. Bronchoalveolar mast cells from asthmatics show enhanced release of mediators such as histamine.

ROLE OF IgE

Most cases of asthma have an allergic background, and allergic processes are regulated by the action of IgE. High levels of serum IgE have been strongly associated with asthma symptoms and with the prevalence of self-reported asthma in patients under the age of 55. In 11-year-old children, asthma prevalence and bronchial hyperresponsiveness have been shown to be related to serum IgE levels. IgE is important for allergen-dependent activation of mast cells, basophils and other inflammatory cells such as eosinophils. Therefore, the cascade of biochemical and molecular events underlying the chronic airways inflammation of asthma may be triggered by interactions between allergens and IgE. The process of sensitization occurs when genetically predisposed individuals are exposed to an allergen. Allergen presentation by immune cells initiates sensitization by inducing a shift of undifferentiated T-helper cells (Th0) towards Th2 phenotype. Th2 lymphocytes secrete interleukins such as IL-4 and IL-13, which induce an isotype switch of B cells to produce IgE. Allergen-specific IgE molecules bind to high-affinity receptors (FcϵRI) on the surface of basophils and mast cells. The antigen-binding regions of IgE are exposed, and binding of an allergen to IgE on the cell surface results in cross-linking and aggregation of IgE receptors, leading to cell degranulation and the release of inflammatory mediators such as histamine, leukotrienes and numerous cytokines. The low-affinity receptor (FcϵRII or CD23) may also mediate the effects of IgE on inflammatory cells such as macrophages and eosinophils. Inhibition of allergic reactions may therefore be achieved by antagonizing the effects of IgE by removing it from the circulation.

EOSINOPHILS AND ASSOCIATED CYTOKINES

The differentiation, bone marrow release, migration into tissues and pathobiological effects of eosinophils occur through the actions of GM-CSF, IL-3, IL-5 and certain chemokines such as eotaxin (Figure 4.7). IL-5 influences the production, maturation, and activation of eosinophils, acting predominantly at the later stages of eosinophil maturation and activation, and can also prolong the survival of eosinophils. IL-5 also causes eosinophils to be released from the bone marrow, while the local release of an eosinophil chemoattractant, such as eotaxin, may be necessary for the tissue localization of eosinophils.

Mature eosinophils may show increased survival in bronchial tissue, secondary to the effects of GM-CSF, IL-3 and IL-5. Eosinophils themselves may also generate other cytokines such as IL-3, IL-5 and GM-CSF. Cytokines such as IL-4 may also exert an important regulatory effect on the expression of adhesion molecules such as VCAM-1, both on endothelial cells of bronchial vessels and on airway epithelial cells. IL-1 and TNFα increase the expression of ICAM-1 or VCAM-1 in both vascular endothelium and airway epithelium.

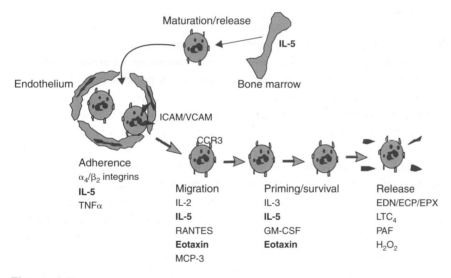

Figure 4.7

The stages leading to eosinophilic inflammation in asthma: from bone marrow release into the circulation, to interactions with the vascular endothelium, migration into the airway mucosa, followed by priming and survival, and activation with release of mediators. ICAM/VCAM, intercellular adhesion molecule/vascular cell adhesion molecule; IL, interleukin; TNF, tumour necrosis factor; RANTES, regulated upon activation, normal T-cell expressed and secreted chemokine; MCP, monocyte chemoattractant protein; GM-CSF, granulocyte/macrophage colony stimulating factor; EDN/ECP/EPX, eosinophil-derived neurotoxin/eosinophil cationic protein/eosinophil protein X; LTC_4, leukotriene C_4; PAF, platelet-activating factor; H_2O_2, hydrogen peroxide.

An anti-IL5 monoclonal antibody administered to mild allergic asthmatics suppressed allergen-induced blood and sputum eosinophilia, without affecting the degree of the late-phase response, indicating that IL-5 may not be the only cytokine involved in allergen-induced late-phase responses.

Eotaxin is a chemoattractant cytokine (chemokine) selective for eosinophils, and acts through the chemokine receptor CCR3 present on eosinophils, basophils and T cells. Cooperation between IL-5 and eotaxin may be necessary for the mobilization of eosinophils from the bone marrow during allergic reactions, and for the local release of chemokines to induce homing and migration into tissues.

Airway wall remodelling

In addition to the chronic cellular inflammation, there are structural changes in the airways of asthmatic patients, often termed airway wall remodelling. These changes include thickening of the airway smooth muscle due to hypertrophy and hyperplasia, myofibroblast activation with increase in subepithelial basement membrane collagen deposition, angiogenesis and increase in submucosal blood vessels and an increase in goblet cell numbers in the airway epithelium (Figure 4.8). These changes may contribute to airway narrowing and bronchial hyperresponsiveness. In addition, it is possible that these may be responsible for the more rapid decline in lung function with age observed in asthmatic patients, and for the impaired therapeutic response to asthma drugs.

The cytokines that have been implicated in the process of airway wall remodelling include the Th2-derived cytokines and growth factors. In genetically modified mice, overexpression of IL-13 in the airway epithelium causes eosinophilic and mononuclear inflammation, with goblet cell hyperplasia, subepithelial fibrosis, airway obstruction and airway hyperresponsiveness, while IL-4, IL-5 and IL-9 overexpression result in substantial mucus metaplasia, and IL-9 and IL-5 overexpression in subepithelial fibrosis and airways hyperresponsiveness. Airway smooth muscle hyperplasia resulted from IL-11 overexpression.

Proliferation of myofibroblasts and the hyperplasia of airway smooth muscle may also occur through the action of several growth factors, such as PDGF and TGFβ, which may be released from inflammatory cells in the airways, such as macrophages and eosinophils. These growth factors may stimulate fibrogenesis by recruiting and activating fibroblasts or transforming myofibroblasts. Epithelial cells may release growth factors, since collagen deposition occurs underneath the basement membrane of the airway epithelium. PDGF and EGF are potent stimulants of human airway smooth muscle proliferation.

Airway smooth muscle cells have the capacity to elaborate a range of cytokines, including IL-4, IL-5, GM-CSF, IL-8, eotaxin and MCP-1, and therefore may play a role in the induction of inflammatory responses

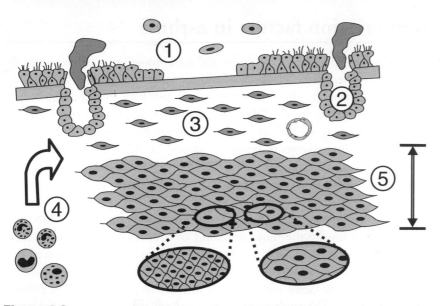

Figure 4.8
Structural remodelling in airways of patients with asthma. (1) Epithelial cell desquamation and disruption; (2) goblet cell hyperplasia and increased secretion of mucus; (3) increased number of fibroblasts with matrix deposition; (4) recruitment of mast cells, T cells and eosinophils; (5) increased airway smooth muscle thickness due to hyperplasia and/or hypertrophy.

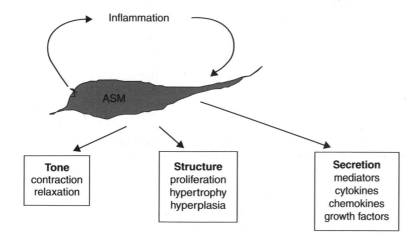

Figure 4.9
The role of the airway smooth muscle (ASM) in asthma and its interaction with the inflammatory process.

(Figure 4.9). Endothelin is another peptide mediator expressed in asthmatic airways that can induce airway smooth muscle, epithelial cell and fibroblast proliferation. In addition, airway smooth muscle cells have the capacity to proliferate under the influence of growth factors, and this accounts for the increased mass of airway smooth muscle observed in asthma.

Transcription factors in asthma

Increased gene expression of cytokines and other proteins in asthma raises the possibility of increased activation of transcription factors that regulate the expression of cytokine genes. Transcription factors play an important role in the long-term regulation of cell function, growth and differentiation. c-Fos, a nuclear proto-oncogene and constituent of the transcriptional activator protein AP-1, has been shown to be overexpressed in the airways epithelium of patients with asthma. Nuclear factor-κB (NF-κB) is another family of transcription factors important in the induction of a wide array of genes, including chemokines, cytokines, enzymes, receptors and stress proteins. It consists of dimeric complexes composed of various members, but the p50/p65 heterodimer is usually the most abundant of the transactivating complexes. NF-κB DNA-binding activity in cells such as macrophages from induced sputum, and in biopsies, of mild asthmatic patients is increased, and the expression of this transcription factor was increased in the airway epithelium of patients with mild asthma. The epithelium in asthma has been shown to be the site of enhanced expression of several proteins, including cytokines such as GM-CSF, RANTES and MCP-1, enzymes such as inducible nitric-oxide synthase (iNOS) and cyclooxygenase (COX)-2, and adhesion molecules such as ICAM-1, and the transcriptional control of these genes is partly dependent on NF-κB activation. A crucial role for NF-κB has been demonstrated in p50(−/−) knock-out mice, which were defective in their capacity to mount an allergic eosinophil response due to lack of production of the Th2 cytokine IL-5 and the chemokine, eotaxin. Other transcription factors of interest in asthma include GATA-3, which is also expressed in the Th2 but not Th1 cells, and is crucial for activation of the IL-5 promoter gene by different stimuli. Ectopic expression of GATA-3 is sufficient to drive IL-5 but not IL-4 gene expression.

Inflammatory mediators in asthma

Many different mediators have been implicated in asthma, possessing a variety of effects on the airways that could account for the pathophysiological features of asthma (Box 4.2). Mediators such as histamine, prostaglandins and leukotrienes contract airway smooth muscle, increase microvascular leakage, cause airway mucus secretion and attract inflammatory cells. Histamine was one of the first mediators implicated in asthma, but its contribution in asthma is unclear, since potent histamine H1-receptor antagonists have not shown any benefit in asthma. It is likely that they do contribute to the pathophysiology of asthma, since combination of a leukotriene antagonist with that of a potent H1-antagonist is more effective in protecting against allergen-induced early

- Histamine
- Sulphidopeptide leukotrienes
- Platelet-activating factor
- Prostaglandins and thromboxane
- Bradykinin
- Adenosine
- Substance P and neurokinin A
- Endothelin
- Nitric oxide
- Reactive oxygen species

Box 4.2
Mediators of asthma

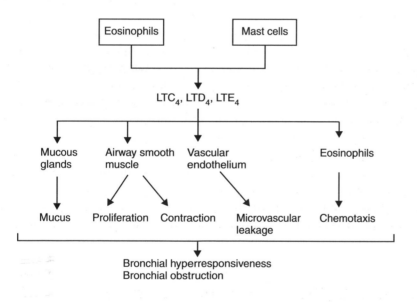

Figure 4.10
Effects of cysteinyl-leukotrienes in asthma.

and late-phase responses than the leukotriene antagonist given alone. The cysteinyl-leukotrienes, LTC_4, LTD_4 and LTE_4, are potent constrictors of human airways and can induce bronchial hyperresponsiveness. Other effects of cysteinyl-leukotrienes have been described, including chemotactic effects on eosinophils and a permissive effect on airway smooth muscle proliferation (Figure 4.10). Potent LTD_4 antagonists protect against exercise- and allergen-induced bronchoconstriction, indicating the contribution of leukotrienes to the bronchoconstrictor responses. Treatment of asthmatic patients with leukotriene receptor antagonists or leukotriene biosynthesis inhibitors improves lung function and symptoms.

Platelet-activating factor (PAF), which is produced by eosinophils and which has pro-inflammatory effects on inflammatory cells such as neutrophils and eosinophils, is also released during asthmatic episodes, such as after exposure to allergen. However, potent PAF receptor antagonists do not provide protection against allergen challenge or benefit to patients with symptomatic asthma.

Products of the cyclooxygenase enzyme pathway include prostaglandins and thromboxane. Prostaglandin (PG) D_2, and $F_{2\alpha}$, and thromboxane may facilitate the release of acetylcholine from cholinergic nerves to augment bronchoconstriction. PGE_2, on the other hand, may have anti-bronchoconstrictor properties and protects against exercise- and allergen-induced bronchoconstriction. Neuropeptides such as substance P, neurokinin A and calcitonin-gene-related peptide may be released from sensitized inflammatory nerves in the airways which increase and extend the ongoing inflammatory response. Neuropeptides may influence immune cells involved in asthma. Thus, neural factors may be important in potentiating bronchoconstriction and inflammation.

Kinins such as bradykinin are generated from $\alpha2$-globulin precursor proteins, kininogens. Bradykinin is generated in the airways following allergen challenge, and also during common viral infections. Bradykinin can cause bronchoconstriction, mucus secretion and plasma exudation in the airways. It activates sensory C-fibres, with concomitant release of neuropeptides, and may therefore enhance neural reflexes in the airways.

Nitric oxide (NO) is produced by the action of enzymes (nitric oxide synthases, NOS), and the increased expression of inducible NOS in the airway epithelium of patients with asthma is likely to underlie the increased levels of NO in exhaled breath. The role of NO as a mediator of asthma remains unclear. Its direct effect as an airway smooth muscle relaxant is small. NO is a potent vasodilator, which may lead to an increase in plasma exudation. It may influence the development of a Th2 response with eosinophilia.

Pathophysiology: the link between inflammation and abnormal physiology

Asthma is characterized by airflow limitation and bronchial hyperresponsiveness, and many of the abnormalities in the airways resulting from chronic inflammatory processes underlie these changes. Airflow limitation may occur through luminal obstruction (such as mucus production and plasma exudation), airway wall oedema and thickening, cellular infiltration and the contractile response of the airway smooth muscle.

Another important abnormality of the airways, bronchial hyperresponsiveness or increased twitchiness of the airways, increases the likelihood of the airways constricting in response to external stimuli such as cold air, exercise or pollutant gases, or to endogenously released bronchoconstrictor mediators such as leukotrienes and histamine. Airway hyperresponsiveness has been characterized not only by an increased likelihood of the airways to constrict in response to low doses of bronchoconstrictor stimuli (airway sensitivity), but also by an excessive amount of narrowing. This excessive narrowing is characterized by the loss of a maximal plateau response at high doses of bronchoconstrictor agent.

The mechanisms underlying the unlimited response during airway smooth muscle contraction are likely to be associated with airways inflammation, particularly the increase in thickness of both muscular and non-muscular components within the airway wall. The degree of airways obstruction will be determined by interactions between airway smooth muscle contraction, airway wall dimensions (thickness), and airway–parenchymal interdependence. The increased amount of airway smooth muscle *per se* may be sufficient to explain excessive airway narrowing, but the oedematous and exudative swelling of the airway wall may augment airway narrowing. Elastic recoil pressure provided by the lung parenchyma is an important determinant of the degree of airway narrowing in small airways, by limiting airway smooth muscle shortening. Peribronchial swelling in asthma may decrease the local parenchymal load, which would lead to excessive airway narrowing. The behaviour of the muscle may also change with the loss of mechanical load in asthma, favouring the development of force-maintenance and preserving very small airway calibre and/or airway closure.

These potential abnormalities of the contractility of the airways have clinical relevance to asthma. In most patients with asthma, airway/parenchymal interdependence is taken advantage of by increasing end-tidal lung volume or by taking a deep inspiration. However, in some patients, loss of bronchodilatation accompanies a deep breath, an effect that has been associated with the amount of airways inflammation and with excessive airway narrowing during bronchoconstriction. This is consistent with the observation that, in severe asthma, there is inflammation of the small airways and of alveoli. In some patients, a deep breath can often lead to severe bronchoconstriction.

Pharmacology and therapy of asthma

5

There is currently no cure for asthma, but with the use of currently available drugs, asthma symptoms are controlled successfully in many patients. In the early 1960s, several drugs became available for treating asthma, including oral theophylline, inhaled and systemic corticosteroids, inhaled sodium cromoglycate, and inhaled and oral β-adrenergic agonists. With the recognition of the role of chronic inflammatory processes in the airways of patients contributing to airway luminal narrowing and bronchial hyperresponsiveness, emphasis has been placed on the regular use of anti-inflammatory therapies such as inhaled corticosteroids. Bronchodilator drugs, such as short-acting inhaled β-agonists, were reserved for intermittent use to relieve any breakthrough symptoms of wheeze or shortness of breath. To emphasize their practical use, anti-inflammatory drugs have also been described as preventors or controllers, and bronchodilator drugs as reliever drugs (Box 5.1). Some drugs may be effective both as a bronchodilator and as an anti-inflammatory drug.

The primary means of achieving control of asthma symptoms is to treat the underlying inflammatory process with anti-inflammatory agents (also called

Bronchodilators (relievers)
- Short-acting β-adrenergic agonists
- Long-acting β-adrenergic agonists
- Slow-release theophylline
- Anticholinergic agents

Anti-inflammatory drugs (preventers or controllers)
- Inhaled corticosteroids
- Oral corticosteroids
- Leukotriene receptor antagonists or leukotriene inhibitors
- Theophylline
- (Long-acting β-agonists)
- (Steroid-sparing agents, e.g. methotrexate, cyclosporin A)

Box 5.1
Classes of drugs for asthma

prophylactic or disease-modifying drugs), particularly inhaled steroids. Early treatment of asthma, such as at the time of diagnosis, can lead to a better improvement in lung function and may prevent the onset of chronic airflow obstruction. Bronchodilators such as β_2-adrenergic agonist drugs, which act mainly by relaxing airway smooth muscle, should be used only for symptomatic relief of airways obstruction. There is no evidence that regular treatment with β_2-adrenergic agonist drugs controls the airway inflammation of asthma. Long-acting β-agonists can now be added to inhaled steroid therapy to provide additional benefits.

Corticosteroids

MODE OF ACTION

Corticosteroid receptors are present in the cytoplasm of most cells, and are rendered active by binding to corticosteroids, which traverse freely through the cell membrane (Figure 5.1). The resulting corticosteroid–corticosteroid

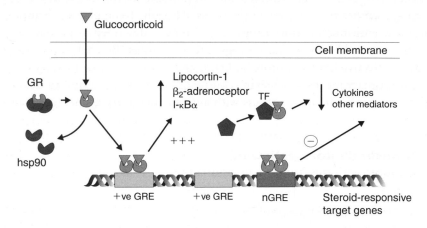

Figure 5.1
Molecular actions of corticosteroids or glucocorticoids. Glucocorticoids bind to their receptor (GR) in the cytoplasm, which leads to the shedding of heat-shock proteins (hsp90). The receptor is thereby activated, and can bind to positive GR elements (GRE) on steroid-responsive target genes to initiate gene transcription of proteins such as lipocortin-1, β_2-adrenoceptors and I-κBα, which may have protective functions in asthma. Activated GR can also bind to negative GREs (nGRE) which can lead to inhibition of gene transcription for certain inflammatory cytokines. Alternatively, activated GR may bind directly to transcription factors (TF) such as NF-κB, and this in turn leads to a reduction in the transcription of pro-inflammatory cytokine genes. The overall effect of glucocorticoids is to cause an inhibition of asthmatic inflammation.

receptor complex is transported to the nucleus, where it binds to specific sequences on the upstream regulatory elements of some genes, leading to increased or decreased protein synthesis. The corticosteroid receptor complex may also bind directly to other proteins, called transcription factors, in the cytoplasm. Transcription factors usually bind to specific sites on genes to activate transcription of certain proteins such as cytokines, and by interfering with the activity of these factors, the steroid–steroid receptor complex can reduce the expression of certain key proteins needed for the inflammation of asthma to be sustained. This action of corticosteroids is independent of an interaction with DNA in the cell nucleus.

These molecular actions of corticosteroids are likely to underlie their suppressive activity on the expression of inflammatory cytokines such as interleukins 4 and 5, GM-CSF, chemokines such as RANTES and eotaxin, and enzymes such as inducible nitric oxide synthase which are overexpressed in asthma. The overall effect of corticosteroids in asthma is to suppress effectively the inflammatory process by inhibition of cytokine and other protein production. Examination of bronchial biopsies obtained from mild asthmatic patients treated with inhaled corticosteroids shows a marked reduction in the number of eosinophils, T-lymphocytes and mast cells, together with a restitution of shed epithelium. Through suppressing certain cytokines such as IL-5 and GM-CSF from cells such as lymphocytes, airway epithelium and monocytes, corticosteroids inhibit the proliferation and differentiation of eosinophil progenitors, and the survival and activation of eosinophils. Corticosteroids suppress the expression of many pro-inflammatory cytokines in T cells and macrophages *in vitro*, including IL-1, IL-2, IL-3, IL-4, IL-5, IL-13 and GM-CSF. They prevent and reverse the increase in microvascular permeability and hence the airway wall oedema seen in asthma, and the secretion of airway mucus from airway submucosal glands. Corticosteroids do not have a direct effect on airway smooth muscle contractility, but prevents the loss of β-adrenoceptor bronchodilator responsiveness induced by inflammatory mediators.

The anti-inflammatory effect of corticosteroids can be demonstrated by inhibition of the late bronchoconstrictor response observed after the inhalation of allergen by allergic asthmatics. This effect represents a suppression of inflammatory cell influx, such as eosinophils and T cells, of cytokine expression and of airway oedema. Treatment with inhaled corticosteroids prevents asthma attacks, particularly nocturnal asthma and exercise-induced asthma. Inhaled steroids have also been associated with a reduction in asthma deaths. Corticosteroids decrease bronchial hyperresponsiveness, which usually reverses by 1–2 doubling doses, but not into the normal range. Clinically, inhaled steroid therapy improves asthma symptoms and lung function such as peak expiratory flow measurements, and reduces diurnal variation in peak flows and the need for relief bronchodilator therapy. Some of the beneficial effects of inhaled steroid therapy are usually observed within a few days of initiating treatment. Discontinuing treatment usually results in the return of asthma symptoms and of bronchial hyperresponsiveness after a variable period of time. Therefore, inhaled corticosteroid therapy does not cure asthma, and the treatment needs to be taken regularly for continued benefit.

PHARMACOKINETICS

Corticosteroids are usually administered by inhalation for the therapy of asthma, but treatment of acute severe attacks necessitates the use of oral or intravenous corticosteroids. The structure of the available topical cortico-steroids in the UK is shown in Figure 5.2. Only 10–20 per cent of the inhaled

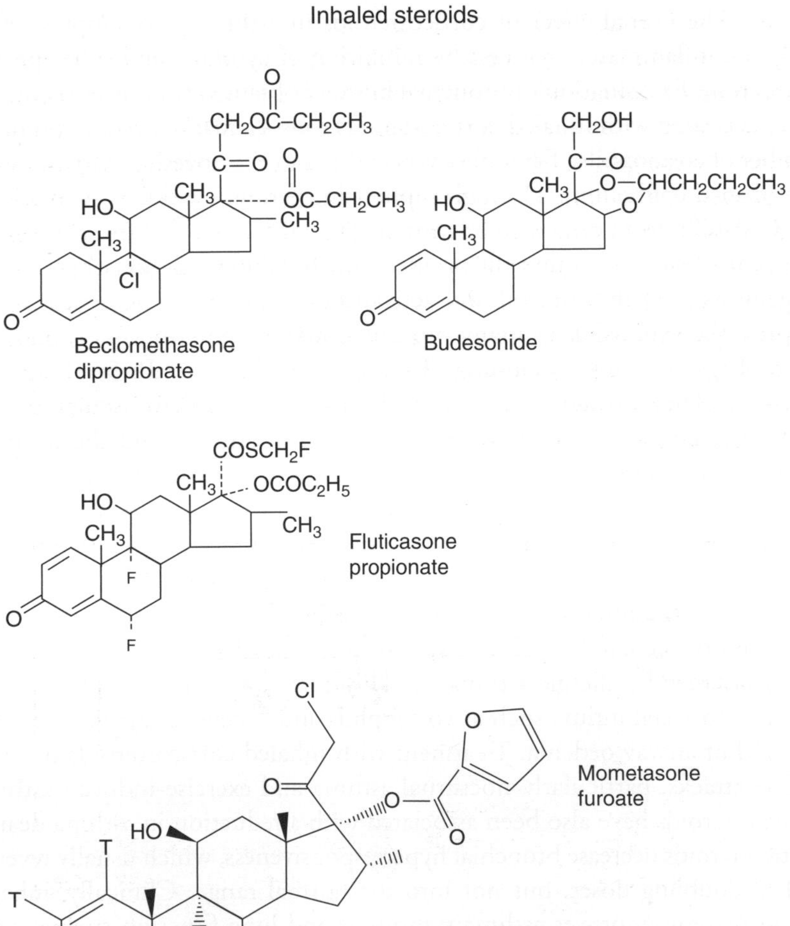

Figure 5.2
Chemical structure of topical corticosteroids which are 16α-, 17α- or 17α, 21α-ester derivatives of hydrocortisone. The ester side-chains are cleaved in the liver, leading to inactivation of the steroid.

Inhaled steroids

Beclomethasone dipropionate

Budesonide

Fluticasone propionate

Mometasone furoate

dose reaches the airways, with the major fraction deposited in the oropharynx where it is swallowed and absorbed from the gut (Figure 5.3). The absorbed fraction is usually metabolized in the liver before reaching the systemic circulation. Oral bioavailability of the newer corticosteroids, such as mometasone furoate and fluticasone propionate, is very low (less than 1 per cent), while that of beclomethasone is 20–30 per cent and that of budesonide is around 11 per cent, reflecting mostly differences in hepatic metabolism. The use of a large-volume spacer device reduces oropharyngeal deposition and therefore can reduce systemic absorption of steroids. The fraction that deposits in the airways is absorbed unchanged into the systemic circulation, since this avoids first-pass metabolism in the liver. Thus, the contribution of airway/lung absorption to systemic effects is potentially greater. Factors such as the potency and affinity for the corticosteroid receptor of the corticosteroid, longer retention in the tissues and release into the bloodstream from the tissues determine the overall systemic contribution.

The residence time of inhaled steroids in the airways, which determines the effectiveness of the steroid, is not known, but this depends on the stability of the steroid and on its lipid solubility. Budesonide and fluticasone propionate are absorbed unchanged from the airways, while beclomethasone dipropionate is converted to the more active beclomethasone monopropionate (BMP) in the airways prior to systemic absorption. The prolonged effect of fluticasone may result from its high lipid solubility, while that of budesonide may be due to the intracellular formation of long-chain fatty acid conjugates which are subsequently released slowly. The potential for systemic effects depends largely on the amount deposited in the airways and absorbed from the airways, on the amount swallowed and escaping first-pass metabolism in the liver and on the relative potency of the steroid.

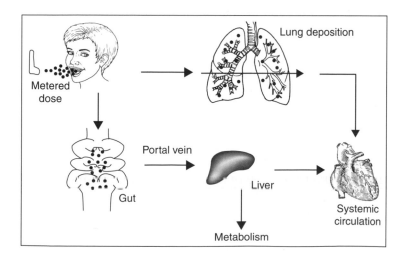

Figure 5.3
Pharmacokinetics of inhaled corticosteroids. The potential systemic effects of inhaled corticosteroids are contributed by (1) the amount of inhaled steroids that deposit in the airways and are absorbed into the systemic circulation, and (2) the amount that is absorbed through the gut and not metabolized in the liver.

CLINICAL USE OF CORTICOSTEROIDS

Inhaled corticosteroids are recommended as first-line therapy for asthma in most countries. In the UK, the British Thoracic Society's (BTS) guidelines advise that this treatment should be instituted in any patient who uses a β-agonist inhaler for symptom control more than three times a week. Treatment is recommended in patients with the mildest asthma symptoms because of demonstrable clinical improvements with inhaled corticosteroid therapy (Box 5.2). Early treatment is also preferable because greater benefit is derived than when treatment is initiated later (Figure 5.4). This reflects the possibility that corticosteroids may be more effective in preventing the structural changes of chronic asthma, than in reversing already-established changes.

The efficacy of steroid aerosols is dose-dependent to some extent, and the dose can be titrated for each patient in order to achieve asthma control, as measured in terms of symptom control, the amount of bronchodilator therapy used, the number of attacks of asthma and the monitoring of peak expiratory flow measurements. However, the dose response for efficacy

Box 5.2
Clinical use of corticosteroids

Effects of corticosteroids on inflammatory processes in asthma
- Reduction in the numbers of mast cells, lymphocytes and eosinophils in the airways.
- Reduction or suppression of the release of mediators from airway macrophages and eosinophils.
- Inhibition of microvascular leakage and oedema.
- Inhibition of cytokine production from lymphocytes (Th2 cells), macrophages and airway epithelium.
- Increase in the number of β_2-receptors on airway smooth muscle and other airway cells.

Clinical benefits of inhaled corticosteroid therapy
- Improves lung function and controls symptoms in patients with mild asthma needing reliever medication on a daily basis.
- Improves lung function and control of symptoms in patients with frequent symptoms and exacerbations.
- Reduces the frequency of exacerbations of asthma.
- Prevents the onset of seasonal asthma symptoms.
- Reduces the need for oral corticosteroid therapy.

(e.g. improvement in PEFR or in bronchial responsiveness) achieves a plateau, usually within the middle range of the recommended inhaled steroid dosages in adult asthmatics with moderately severe asthma. The steroid dose–response curve may also vary according to the severity of asthma. It may be preferable to start with a relatively high dose of inhaled corticosteroids to effectively control the symptoms in a patient with more severe asthma. Once under control after a period of 2–3 months, the dose of inhaled steroids can be titrated down to a maintenance dose. This is a step that is often forgotten. Overall, most patients with asthma achieve the best benefit at doses of inhaled steroids of the order of 800–1000 μg of beclomethasone or equivalent.

In patients with more severe asthma, the dose of inhaled corticosteroids may be increased to the maximum recommended doses, but this should be performed under supervision so that any lack of efficacy can be followed by a reduction of the dose. Adding a long-acting β-agonist, theophylline or a leukotriene inhibitor may be as effective or provide better control than

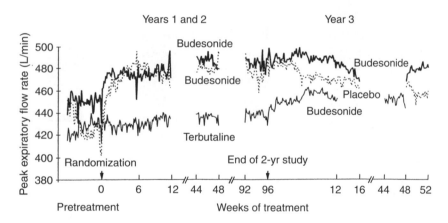

Figure 5.4
Effect of treatment with inhaled corticosteroids (budesonide) compared to a β-agonist (terbutaline) on morning peak expiratory flow rate (PEFR) in newly diagnosed mild asthmatic patients. In the two groups of patients receiving budesonide during the first 2 years, there was an improvement in PEFR which was maintained, while the terbutaline-treated group showed no change in PEFR. During the third year, one group that had been treated with budesonide switched to placebo, with subsequent worsening of PEFR, while the terbutaline-treated group switched to budesonide. In the latter group, the PEFR improvement was not as large as that of the groups that were treated with budesonide during the first 2 years. This study indicates that early treatment with inhaled corticosteroids gives the greatest beneficial effects. (Reprinted with permission from Haahtela *et al.* (1991) *N. Engl. J. Med.* **325**, 388–92.)

increasing doses of inhaled corticosteroids. In a minority of patients, further control of asthma may be obtained by addition of regular oral corticosteroids, and the patient may become 'corticosteroid-dependent'.

Inhaled corticosteroids are usually administered twice daily, either from a metered-dose inhaler (MDI) or from a powder inhaler. A volume-spacer device in conjunction with MDIs is recommended, particularly when high doses of inhaled steroids are used, in order to ensure a higher amount of lung deposition compared with lesser deposition in the throat and larynx (see p. 92). In patients with mild to moderately severe asthma, a single daily dose of inhaled corticosteroid (e.g. budesonide or mometasone) may be effective in controlling asthma, which may help to improve adherence to treatment.

Figure 5.5
(a) Rate of severe exacerbations of asthma in patients treated with budesonide 200 μg twice daily or 800 μg twice daily (BUD200 or BUD800), or with combined therapy of budesonide and formoterol (BUD200+F or BUD800+F). The higher dose of budesonide was effective in reducing the exacerbation rate, while addition of formoterol at each dose of budesonide had an inhibitory effect on these rates.
(b) Changes in peak expiratory flow rates (PEF) in these four groups, demonstrating the persistent bronchodilator response due to the addition of formoterol over the 12-month period. (Reprinted with permission from Pauwels *et al.* (1997) *N. Engl. J. Med.* **337**, 1405–11. Copyright © 1997 Massachusetts Medical Society.)

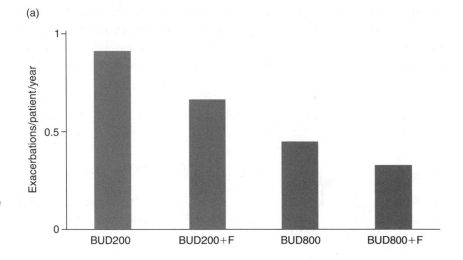

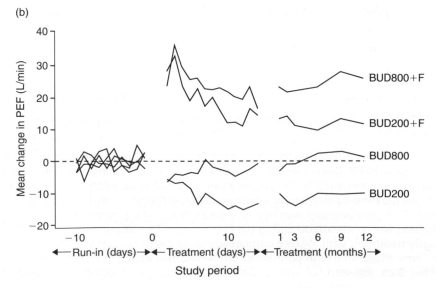

Corticosteroids (budesonide and fluticasone propionate) in the nebulized formulation are available and have been recommended for use in patients with severe asthma, often as an oral corticosteroid-sparing agent. Very high doses can be administered in this way. There is little evidence to support their use in this situation, and this has not been shown to be any superior to administration of the same corticosteroids delivered from a conventional hand-held inhaler.

Inhaled corticosteroids reduce the occurrence of exacerbations of asthma (Figure 5.5). In patients already on inhaled corticosteroids, it is often recommended that they double their dose at the onset of an exacerbation, although there is no convincing evidence that this will curb the exacerbation. High-dose inhaled steroids may hasten recovery from an exacerbation of asthma, but this treatment cannot be recommended for the treatment of acute severe asthma. Short courses of oral corticosteroids, such as prednisolone 40 mg/day for 10 days, are indicated for exacerbations of asthma. Usually, it is recommended that the dose of 40 mg/day should be continued until symptoms have improved and peak flow measurements have returned to their usual values, followed by a gradual tapering and stopping the treatment. With more severe asthma associated with respiratory failure or gastrointestinal upsets, intravenous hydrocortisone (100–200 mg 6–8 hourly) is recommended.

CURRENTLY AVAILABLE INHALED CORTICOSTEROIDS

Several inhaled corticosteroids are available (Table 5.1): beclomethasone dipropionate, budesonide and fluticasone propionate are inhaled from metered dose inhalers and from multidose dry-powder inhalers. More recently, mometasone furoate has been introduced and is only available as a multidose dry-powder inhaler. With the abolition of chlorofluorocarbon (CFC) propellants, hydrofluorocarbon (HFC) propellants are now being use in metered-dose inhalers. An HFC-beclomethasone is now available and its lung deposition is twice that of CFC-beclomethasone. Budesonide and fluticasone are also available as nebulized suspensions.

The recommended dose ranges for adults are as follows: beclomethasone dipropionate 200–2000 μg/day, budesonide 200–1600 μg/day, fluticasone 100–1000 μg/day and mometasone 200–800 μg/day. The clinical potency of beclomethasone is the weakest, while those of fluticasone and mometasone are superior to that of budesonide. In mild to moderate asthma, once-daily dosing of budesonide or of mometasone appears to be as effective as twice-daily dosing in terms of improvement in lung function, which is helpful in maintaining adherence to treatment. However, in more severe asthma, a twice-daily dosing is needed.

At high doses of budesonide, fluticasone and mometasone, fewer systemic effects are encountered, due to the increased first-pass hepatic metabolism of

Table 5.1
Inhaled corticosteroid preparations

Generic name	Brand name	Breath-actuated with integral drug	Breath-actuated device with drug	MDI with integral spacer	MDI alone	MDI plus separate spacer	Nebulizer solution
Beclomethasone dipropionate	Aerobec	Autohaler					No
	Asmabec	Clickhaler					
	Beclazone				MDI		
	Becloforte	Easi-breathe	Diskhaler and disks		MDI	Volumatic	
	Becodisks		Diskhaler and Becodisks				
	Becotide	Easi-breathe	Rotahaler and Rotacaps		MDI	Volumatic	
	Filair	Autohaler			MDI		
	Qvar	Autohaler			MDI	Aerochamber	
Budesonide	Pulmicort	Turbohaler		Spacer adapter	MDI	Nebuhaler	Yes
Budesonide with formoterol	Symbicort	Turbohaler					
Fluticasone propionate	Flixotide	Accuhaler	Diskhaler and disks		MDI Evohaler (CFC-free)	Volumatic	Yes
Fluticasone with salmeterol	Seretide	Accuhaler			Evohaler (CFC-free)	Volumatic	
Mometasone furoate	Asmanex	Twisthaler					

MDI, Metered dose inhaler; CFC, chlorofluorocarbon.

these corticosteroids. The type of delivery device used is important in comparing different types of corticosteroids, since each manufacturer has its own type of inhaler device for its products. Overall, therefore, many criteria are needed in the assessment in the choice of the 'best' corticosteroid for a particular type of patients, including the type of patient that the prescription is for, the severity of the asthma, the inhaler device, the dose of corticosteroid envisaged, the therapeutic: side-effect ratio and the cost implications. Such assessment is difficult because of the lack of studies that have combined both efficacy and systemic bioavailability outcomes over a range of doses, not only on the flat part of the dose–response curve.

SIDE-EFFECTS

Inhaled corticosteroids are usually well tolerated. Side-effects can be divided into local and systemic groups. Local side-effects are accounted for by the deposition of corticosteroids in the oropharyngeal spaces, while potential systemic side-effects arise from the systemic availability of absorption from the deposited corticosteroid in the airways and lungs, and from the fraction absorbed into the hepato-portal circulation that escapes first-pass hepatic metabolism (Box 5.3).

Oral treatment
- Adrenal suppression
- Growth suppression
- Bruising
- Osteoporosis
- Cataracts
- Glaucoma
- Metabolic disturbances
- Psychiatric disturbances

Inhaled
- Adrenal suppression (high doses)
- Growth suppression (high doses)
- Bruising
- Reduced bone density
- Cataracts
- Local: dysphonia, oropharyngeal candidiasis

Box 5.3
Side-effects of corticosteroid therapy

Local

Dysphonia and weakness of voice, leading to loss of voice, is secondary to a localized laryngeal myopathy and is not an uncommon complaint, particularly amongst those who use their voice professionally (e.g. singers, teachers and lecturers). A smaller number (~5 per cent) develop oropharyngeal candidiasis, particularly those on high-dose steroids. The incidence of local side-effects can be reduced by teaching the patient proper instructions of inhaler technique and by the use of a volume-spacer device and by mouth-rinsing after inhalation. Antifungal agents may be needed to control local symptoms of candidiasis, without the need to discontinue inhaled corticosteroids. Often, a reduction in the dose of inhaled steroids leads to an improvement in dysphonia.

Systemic

The systemic side-effects of chronic administration of oral corticosteroids are well documented. These include fluid retention, weight gain due to increased appetite, osteoporosis, skin bruising, hypertension, cataracts, diabetes, peptic ulceration and psychosis. Biochemical evidence of systemic side-effects can usually be obtained at high doses of inhaled steroids, although there is variability between preparations. The clinical relevance of these abnormal biochemical tests remains to be determined.

Adrenal suppression

Mild suppression of basal endogenous cortisol secretion by normal therapeutic doses of inhaled corticosteroids is unlikely to be important. Biochemical evidence of adrenal suppression rarely occurs with dosages below 1000 μg daily of beclomethasone or budesonide in adults. In children, doses of beclomethasone dipropionate up to 800 μg/day over a period of 2–5 years does not appear to affect the hypothalamo-pituitary–adrenal axis. Differences between available inhaled corticosteroids are controversial. Greater adrenal suppression with beclomethasone than with equi-effective doses of budesonide or fluticasone has been described. Fluticasone had the greatest potential for systemic side-effects on the hypothalamo-pituitary axis, particularly at doses above 800 μg/day, in normal subjects, but in asthmatics, much less significant effects are observed. This may be explained by the fact that, following inhalation, normal non-asthmatic subjects absorb twice as much fluticasone as patients with asthma. No suppression of the hypothalamo-pituitary axis has been observed following administration of the clinically recommended doses of mometasone furoate between 200 and 800 μg/day. Some suppression is observed at a dose of 1600 μg/day.

Effects on bone

Biochemical markers of bone turnover, such as serum osteocalcin and urinary hydroxyproline, can be increased by inhaled steroids in adults, usually at high doses. Studies of small groups of asthmatics found no detrimental effects on bone mineral density, measured by dual X-ray absorptiometry in children receiving becomethasone, budesonide or fluticasone at the conventional doses for 2–6 years. The clinical significance of these observations with regard to the development of osteoporosis, particularly in premenopausal women, is not known. There is no current evidence that inhalation of corticosteroids is associated with increased risk of osteoporosis or fractures in children or adults.

Effects on growth

Some studies in children using doses of beclomethasone of 200–900 μg/day, budesonide up to 400 μg/day (via MDI plus spacer or Turbohaler®), or fluticasone 200 μg/day (via MDI plus spacer) did not have adverse effects on growth. However, more recent studies have shown a slowing of growth with beclomethasone 400 μg by MDI or dry powder. Using a short-term measure of the linear growth of the lower leg, knemometry, a reduction in growth can be demonstrated with medium doses of inhaled corticosteroids; however, the significance of this is unclear. In recent large studies on growth in asthmatic children (5–9 years) treated with budesonide at doses ~400 μg/day, a 20 per cent fall in growth velocity during the first year of treatment was observed but growth subsequently recovered, and the children attained normal adult height. On the other hand, inhaled steroids can improve growth by improving asthma, since chronic uncontrolled asthma may itself cause stunting. Growth suppression can certainly occur if very high doses of corticosteroids (e.g. >1000 μg fluticasone daily) are inhaled, and may even occur in some individuals at 'normal' therapeutic doses. It is therefore important to monitor growth in any children on chronic inhaled corticosteroid therapy; those with a high maintenance dose should be reviewed regularly by a paediatrician.

Other effects

Other systemic effects, such as dermal thinning and easy skin bruising and an increased incidence of subcapsular cataract formation, have been reported in elderly asthmatics, although many of these patients have also taken short courses of oral prednisolone. In a group of children treated with budesonide (mean dose 504 μg/day), there was no increased risk of posterior subcapsular cataract, bruising or voice changes, compared to a group of asthmatics not exposed to inhaled corticosteroids.

Sodium cromoglycate and nedocromil sodium

Sodium cromoglycate is a synthetic bischromone derivative of the Egyptian herbal plant khellin, and was one of the earlier inhaled drugs to be used for the prophylaxis and prevention of asthma attacks. Its anti-asthma effects were discovered when it was found to inhibit the early and late-phase bronchoconstrictor response to allergen. Nedocromil sodium is a related compound, the sodium salt of pyranoquinolone dicarboxylic acid, with similar properties to sodium cromoglycate.

MODE OF ACTION

Sodium cromoglycate was developed initially as a mast-cell stabilizer, and, together with nedocromil sodium, it inhibits the IgE-mediated release of histamine from human lung mast cells. Nedocromil sodium is more potent than sodium cromoglycate in this respect. Both agents act on other anti-inflammatory cells. Sodium cromoglycate and nedocromil sodium also inhibit some aspect of activation of the eosinophil and the macrophage. Both inhaled drugs can prevent the immediate early (mediated by mast cells) and the late (involving T cells and eosinophils) responses observed following allergen challenge in allergic asthmatics. Sodium cromoglycate also reduces the seasonal increases in bronchial responsiveness in asthmatic subjects with grass pollen sensitivity. Nedocromil sodium prevents the deterioration in asthma in steroid-dependent asthmatics undergoing a reduction in inhaled steroid dosage. However, studies of bronchial biopsies in asthmatics demonstrate a small decrease in the influx of eosinophils after treatment with nedocromil sodium. Other actions of these drugs include inhibition of bronchoconstriction induced by agents that are believed to act through activation of airway sensory nerves, such as sulphur dioxide, sodium metabisulphite and bradykinin, with nedocromil sodium being more potent than sodium cromoglycate. These drugs may inhibit activation of neural mechanisms in the airways, such as the induction of cough. Both drugs may work at a molecular level by blocking a specific chloride channel in various cells, including mast cells, airway epithelial cells and sensory nerves. In summary, sodium cromoglycate and nedocromil sodium have preventive, anti-inflammatory effects, without affecting airway smooth muscle tone.

PHARMACOKINETICS

Because of its poor absorption through mucous membranes, only a small proportion of inhaled sodium cromoglycate can be detected in the circulation, the amount depending on inspiratory flow rate. Peak plasma levels are achieved within 15–20 min of inhalation. Sodium cromoglycate is secreted unchanged in bile and urine. Nedocromil sodium is absorbed to a limited extent when taken orally, and only 5–10 per cent of an inhaled dose is absorbed primarily from the respiratory tract. No metabolism is detected and plasma clearance is rapid.

CLINICAL USE

Sodium cromoglycate and nedocromil sodium are used as prophylaxis, and are particularly effective in preventing asthma attacks induced by exposure to allergens or following exercise. It is likely that atopic patients respond better. These drugs are indicated in asthmatics, particularly children, whose symptoms are not well controlled by a β-agonist inhaler alone. In a crossover study, nedocromil sodium was more effective than regular salbutamol in improving daytime asthma symptoms, wheezing and shortness of breath. The effects of nedocromil have been compared to those of low-dose beclomethasone dipropionate (400 μg/day) in terms of symptom control. However, in a large study in children, nedocromil sodium had very little effect on asthma control as measured by hospitalizations, urgent visits for medical help, courses of prednisolone and need for salbutamol. A recent systematic review of all published randomized, placebo-controlled trials of sodium cromoglycate in the prophylactic treatment of children with asthma found insufficient evidence that this drug has a beneficial effect.

Both sodium cromoglycate (10 mg four times daily via MDI or spinhaler, to a maintenance dose of 5 mg four times daily) and nedocromil sodium (4 mg four times daily via MDI to a maintenance dose of 4 mg twice a day) should be used daily over a trial period of 4 weeks. If there is no effect on asthma control, inhaled corticosteroid therapy should be used.

SIDE-EFFECTS

Sodium cromoglycate is remarkably devoid of side-effects, except for transient coughing and throat irritation. These can usually be prevented by prior administration of a β-agonist inhaler. The main side-effects with nedocromil sodium include a distinctive bitter taste, nausea and headache. A menthol-flavoured preparation may overcome the bitter taste.

Anti-leukotrienes

A new class of anti-asthma drugs, the anti-leukotrienes, have recently been introduced for the treatment of asthma. In the UK, drugs that block the leukotriene receptor have become available. An inhibitor of leukotriene synthesis can also be prescribed in the USA.

MODE OF ACTION

Leukotriene receptor antagonists inhibit the effects of cysteinyl-leukotrienes released during asthma attacks. Cysteinyl-leukotrienes can be detected in bronchoalveolar lavage fluid and in the urine of patients with asthma. They comprise LTC_4, LTD_4 and LTE_4, and are generated in inflammatory cells from arachidonic acid by the enzyme, 5-lipoxygenase. They are potent bronchoconstrictors, cause microvascular leakage and oedema of the airway wall, and stimulate airway mucus secretion, in addition to causing eosinophil chemotaxis into the airways. These effects are mediated through the cys-LT1 receptor, and several antagonists of the cys-LT1 receptor have been developed. In addition, inhibitors of the 5-lipoxygenase enzymes have been developed, such as zileuton. These drugs may be considered as anti-inflammatory.

Antagonists of cys-LT1 receptor include zafirlukast, pranlukast and montelukast. They prevent bronchoconstriction induced by inhaled cysteinyl-leukotrienes, in addition to that induced by allergen, exercise and cold air. Aspirin-induced bronchoconstriction in aspirin-induced asthmatics is also inhibited. Leukotriene inhibitors also reduce eosinophilic inflammation in the airways.

CLINICAL USE

In several clinical studies, leukotriene receptor antagonists caused bronchodilatation, implying that leukotrienes contribute to baseline bronchoconstriction in asthma. Leukotriene receptor antagonists are effective in inhibiting exercise-induced asthma, and in preventing early and late-phase responses after allergen. An increase in peak flow measurements, a reduction in β_2-agonist usage and an improvement in symptom scores in moderately severe asthma have been observed (Figure 5.6). Such improvements are obtained in patients who are not on inhaled steroids, as well as those who are already taking such therapy. Leukotriene receptor antagonists also provide additional control when added to inhaled corticosteroid therapy, in patients in whom corticosteroid therapy is not entirely effective. In patients with more severe asthma, they may reduce asthma exacerbation rates and improve lung function, and may allow for a reduction in oral or inhaled corticosteroid dose. Similar to the response to inhaled corticosteroid therapy, the beneficial responses vary between patients and the factors or features that determines good responses are not known.

Two oral leukotriene receptor antagonists are available in the UK: montelukast for adults and children older than 6 years, and zafirlukast for adults and children older than 12 years. The use of these leukotriene receptor antagonists in the management of asthma is not definitely established. They could be used for the management of mild, moderate and severe asthma. For the mild asthmatic, leukotriene receptor antagonists may be used as first-line treatment, but they are less efficacious than low-dose inhaled corticosteroids. Leukotriene receptor antagonists have the advantage of being in the form of

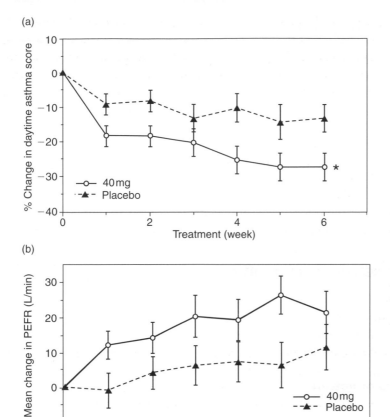

(a)

(b)

Figure 5.6
Effect of a cysteinyl-
leukotriene receptor
antagonist (zafirlukast or
Accolate®, 20 mg twice
per day) on daytime
asthma score
(a) and on peak
expiratory flow rate
(PEFR) (b) in patients
with mild to moderately
severe asthma.
(Reprinted with
permission from Spector
et al. (1994) *Am. J.
Respir. Crit. Care Med.*
150, 618–32.)

an oral tablet; patients may adhere more to this therapy than to use of a corticosteroid inhaler. In addition, patients are less concerned about potential
corticosteroid side-effects. Leukotriene receptor antagonists may be added to
moderate doses of inhaled corticosteroids for additional control of asthma, or
to higher doses of inhaled or oral corticosteroids in severe asthma. A therapeutic trial for 1 month is usually recommended before establishing the
patient on the treatment.

Leukotriene receptor antagonists are generally well tolerated and there are
no serious side-effects. Common side-effects include headaches, nausea and
vomiting, gastrointestinal upsets, skin rashes and occasional abnormalities of
liver function tests. A few cases of Churg–Strauss syndrome, characterized by
systemic vasculitis with eosinophilia and asthma, have been observed in
patients on zafirlukast and montelukast. It is unclear whether this is due to a
reduction in oral corticosteroids, allowing the vasculitis to flare up, or
whether this is a direct effect of the drug.

Bronchodilators

Bronchodilator drugs have an anti-bronchoconstrictor effect and cause immediate reversal of airways obstruction in asthma patients due to a primary effect on airway smooth muscle. Three types of bronchodilators are in current clinical use:

- β_2-adrenergic agonists (sympathomimetics);
- methylxanthines (theophylline);
- anticholinergic drugs (ipratropium bromide/oxitropium bromide).

Leukotriene inhibitors have bronchodilator effects by inhibiting the bronchoconstrictor effects of leukotrienes and are described above.

β-ADRENERGIC AGONISTS

Inhaled β_2-agonists are the most effective bronchodilators available, with an immediate onset of action associated with minimal side-effects. Two types are now available: short-acting over 3–4 hours and long-acting over 12 hours. Their structure is shown in Figure 5.7.

Mode of action
β-Agonists produce bronchodilatation by direct stimulation of β_2-receptors in airway smooth muscle, leading to relaxation. β-Receptors have been demonstrated in airway smooth muscle of all airways from the trachea to the terminal bronchioles. Binding of β_2-agonist to the β_2-receptor leads to activation of adenylate cyclase, which increases intracellular cyclic adenosine $3',5'$-monophosphate, leading in turn to activation of protein kinase A (Figure 5.8). This enzyme phosphorylates several proteins in the cell, leading to lowering of intracellular calcium ions and to inhibition of myosin light-chain kinase, and ultimately to relaxation of the airway smooth muscle. Other important effects of β_2-receptor activation include the opening of a potassium channel in the cell membrane, which may lead to relaxation of the muscle.

β-Agonists act as functional antagonists and reverse bronchoconstriction irrespective of the contractile agent. β-Agonists may have additional effects on airways, including: (1) prevention of mediator release from lung mast cells; (2) reduction of airway microvascular leakage and oedema; (3) reduction of neurotransmission of cholinergic nerves; and (4) increased mucus production from airway submucosal glands. The relevance of these additional effects with chronic treatment is not known, but the rapid bronchodilator effect of β-agonists is likely to be attributable to a direct effect on airway smooth muscle. It is unlikely that β-agonists possess any significant anti-inflammatory effects in asthma.

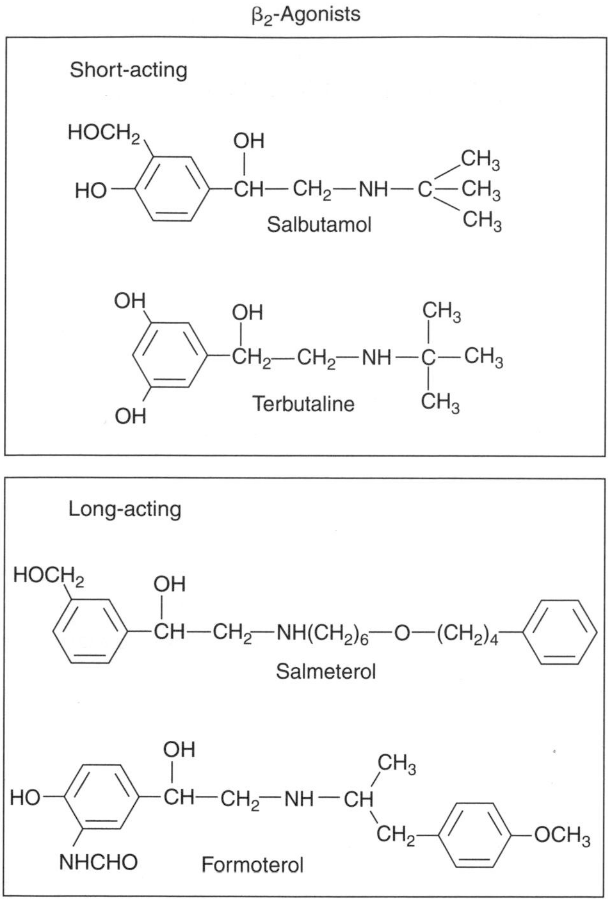

β$_2$-Agonists

Short-acting

Salbutamol

Terbutaline

Long-acting

Salmeterol

Formoterol

Figure 5.7
Chemical structure of short-acting and long-acting β-adrenergic agonists in clinical use.

Clinical use

Short-acting β-agonists inhaled from a metered-dose inhaler or from a dry-powder inhaler are the most widely used bronchodilators in mild exacerbations. In acute severe asthma, the nebulized route of administration is as effective as the intravenous route. For chronic use, it is recommended that β-agonists are used only for breakthrough symptoms as necessary. Increased usage is usually taken as an indicator of loss of control, and of the need to use more anti-inflammatory treatment. Some patients need to use regular β-agonists, and studies have now shown that there is no risk of worsening asthma as a result of this.

Although slow-release oral preparations of short-acting β-agonists may be used for the control of nocturnal asthma in children, these are much less effective than inhaled β-agonists, particularly long-acting β-agonists.

Long-acting β-agonists, such as salmeterol and formoterol, have a bronchodilator and protective effect of more than 12 hours, and are particularly

Figure 5.8
Molecular actions of β-adrenoceptor agonists to cause airway smooth muscle relaxation. The seven-transmembrane β-receptor is activated on binding to a β-agonist, leading to adenylate cyclase activation through coupling with a stimulatory G protein (G_s). Adenylate cyclase catalyses the formation of cyclic adenosine monophosphate (cAMP), which leads to activation of protein kinase A. This protein phosphorylates a number of other proteins that lead to airway smooth muscle relaxation. cAMP is metabolized to 5'-AMP by phosphodiesterase (PDE) isoenzymes.

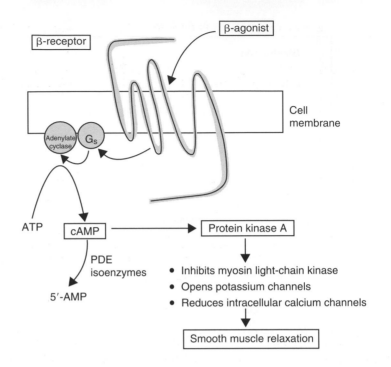

Figure 5.9
Duration of the effect of the long-acting β-agonist, salmeterol. Mean FEV_1 response in patients with asthma following inhalation of salmeterol (42 μg twice daily) or of salbutamol (180 μg four times daily), showing the sustained bronchodilator response over 12 hours with salmeterol, without development of tolerance. (Reproduced with permission from Pearlman *et al.* (1992) *N. Engl. J. Med.* **327**, 1420–5. Copyright © 1992 Massachusetts Medical Society.)

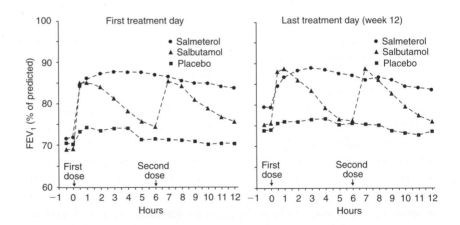

useful in the control of nocturnal asthma (Figure 5.9). These β-agonists provide improved asthma control when administered twice daily, compared to four times daily for a short-acting β-agonist. When introduced to patients not controlled on either 400 or 800 μg inhaled beclomethasone dipropionate, salmeterol provided better control of asthma compared to an increased dose of inhaled corticosteroid, both in adults and children (Figure 5.10). Similar results have been found with formoterol, which has also been shown to reduce the frequency of exacerbations (Figure 5.5). Therefore, one clinical

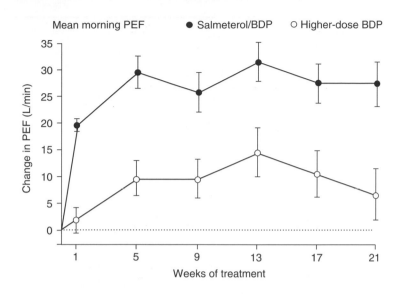

Figure 5.10
Effect of adding salmeterol to a low dose of inhaled corticosteroids (beclomethasone dipropionate, BDP, 200 µg twice daily) compared to increasing the dose of BDP to 500 µg twice daily on morning peak expiratory flow (PEF). There was a better effect of the combination therapy on PEF than the higher dose of inhaled BDP. (Reprinted with permission from Elsevier Science from Greening *et al.* (1994) *The Lancet* **344**, 219–24.)

use of long-acting β-agonists is to combine them with low to medium doses of inhaled corticosteroids in patients not adequately controlled on inhaled steroids alone. It is currently recommended that long-acting β-agonists not be used as monotherapy of asthma, since their long duration of action may mask worsening airway inflammation.

The long-acting β-agonist, formoterol, may be used safely as a reliever bronchodilator, with greater effectiveness than salbutamol.

Choice of β-agonist

The two most-commonly used specific β_2-adrenergic agonist are salbutamol and terbutaline (Table 5.2), with a duration of bronchodilator effect of 3–4 hours. Other short-acting β_2-agonists in clinical use are fenoterol and reproterol. There is probably little to choose between the various preparations at the current recommended doses. Higher doses of fenoterol have been used previously. The preferred mode of administration is either by a metered-dose inhaler or a powder inhaler (Table 5.2). Larger amounts can be delivered from a nebulizer, as used for the treatment of acute severe asthma. Oral slow-release preparations of salbutamol and terbutaline are available, and are usually associated with more systemic side-effects than inhaled therapy. Bambuterol is a pro-drug of terbutaline and has a sustained bronchodilator effect, lasting up to 24 hours when taken orally. These oral preparations are less efficacious than the inhaled ones. Inhaled β_2-agonists with a long duration of action (over 12 hours), such as formoterol and salmeterol, are suitable for twice-daily dosing. Formoterol has a more rapid onset of action and is a fuller agonist than salmeterol, the clinical significance of this observation is not known.

Table 5.2
Inhaled β-agonist bronchodilators

Generic name	Brand name	Breath-actuated with integral drug	Breath-actuated with drug	MDI with spacer	MDI alone	MDI with separate spacer	Nebulizer solution
Short-acting							
Fenoterol	Berotec				MDI		
Fenoterol and ipratropium	Duovent	Autohaler			MDI		
Reproterol	Bronchodil				MDI		
Salbutamol	Aerolin	Autohaler					
	Airomir	Autohaler					
	Asmasal	Clickhaler					
	Salamol			Spacehaler	MDI		Yes
	Salbulin				MDI	Aerochamber	
	Ventodisks		Diskhaler and ventodisks				
	Ventolin	(1) Accuhaler (2) Easi-breathe	Rotahaler and rotacaps		Evohaler	Volumatic	Yes
Salbutamol and ipratropium	Combivent			Spacer inhaler	MDI		Yes
Terbutaline	Bricanyl	Turbohaler			MDI	Nebuhaler	Yes
Long-acting							
Formoterol	Foradil		Inhaler and capsules				
	Oxis	Turbohaler					
Salmeterol	Serevent	Accuhaler	Diskhaler and disks		MDI	Volumatic	

Tolerance to the bronchodilator and bronchoprotective effects of these long-acting β-agonists has been demonstrated, but is not likely to be of any clinical significance.

Combined preparations of inhaled corticosteroids and long-acting β-agonists are now available, usually administered twice daily (for example, the combination of fluticasone propionate and salmeterol, and that of budesonide and formoterol). These are convenient for patients needing both therapies and may help to improve adherence to treatment. In addition, when taken together, the combination has greater beneficial effects than when taken separately, indicating some synergistic beneficial effects.

Side-effects

Side-effects are not common with inhaled therapy, but are more common with oral or intravenous administration. Muscle tremor due to stimulation of β_2-receptors in skeletal muscle, tachycardia and palpitations are the most common side-effects. Metabolic side-effects such as hypokalaemia are usually observed after large systemic doses, and may be important when treating acute severe asthma. The combination of hypokalaemia and hypoxaemia may predispose to cardiac dysrhythmias.

Tolerance to β-agonists

Tolerance to the effect of β-agonists with prolonged use has been described on airway smooth muscle studied *in vitro*. Although bronchodilator tolerance has been described in normal subjects after high doses of inhaled salbutamol, no such tolerance has been observed in patients with mild asthma. There appears to be no tolerance to the bronchodilator effect of salmeterol, but tolerance to the bronchoprotective effects of short-acting and long-acting β-agonists has been described, but is not clinically significant since bronchoprotection is still present. Inhaled corticosteroids may not protect against tolerance to the bronchoprotective effects of inhaled β-agonists.

Safety studies

The rise in asthma deaths in the early 1960s, and in New Zealand in the 1980s, have been linked to the excessive use of β-agonists. In New Zealand, this association was strengthened by the observation of a fall in asthma mortality when the β-agonist, fenoterol, was removed from the market. Further studies have also implicated the chronic use of fenoterol with loss of control of asthma. However, more recent studies with regular salbutamol have not confirmed this, and it is likely that the previous association of β-agonist usage with rising asthma deaths reflected a group of patients with severe asthma at high risk of asthma death. What is not known is whether excessive use of short-acting β-agonists (say more than 12 puffs per 24 hours) is deleterious, and it would make sense to reduce such excessive use. There is no evidence that long-acting β-agonists, used twice daily over up to 1 year, has any deleterious effects on asthma control, provided that concomitant inhaled corticosteroid therapy is established.

Clinical use

β_2-Agonists are the most widely used and effective bronchodilators in the treatment of asthma. When inhaled from metered-dose aerosols, they are convenient and easy to use, rapid in onset and without significant side-effects. In addition to an acute bronchodilator effect, they are effective in protecting against various challenges, such as exercise, cold air and allergen. They are the bronchodilators of choice in the treatment of acute severe asthma, where the nebulized route of administration is as effective as the intravenous use. The inhaled route of administration is preferable to the oral route because side-effects are fewer, and also because it may be more effective.

β-Agonists do not have significant anti-inflammatory effects in asthma, unlike steroids. Short-acting β-agonists should therefore be used for symptom control and should not be given as regular therapy to control asthma symptoms, unless concomitant anti-inflammatory or prophylactic treatment is also prescribed. Increased usage of short-acting β_2-agonists indicates the need for more anti-inflammatory therapy. Long-acting β_2-agonists, such as salmeterol, should be administered to patients already established on inhaled corticosteroid therapy. A minimum dose of 400–800 μg/day of inhaled beclomethasone or equivalent has been recommended prior to addition of long-acting β_2-agonist therapy, which may be useful in controlling persistent nocturnal, early morning or daytime wheeze.

THEOPHYLLINE

Theophylline has been used widely for the treatment of asthma since 1930, and is one of the most common treatments worldwide. Improvements in slow-release preparations and the availability of rapid plasma assays for theophylline levels have further strengthened its use. Theophylline is a bronchodilator and also possesses some anti-inflammatory effects, in modulating eosinophil and T-cell inflammation. However, its efficacy in both instances is rather limited. In addition, many patients cannot tolerate its side-effects of headaches and nausea.

Mode of action

The mechanism of action of theophylline in asthma remains unclear. Many proposed mechanisms do not explain its effects entirely. It has been proposed that it may act as an inhibitor of phosphodiesterases which break down cyclic

AMP in the cell, leading to an increase in cellular concentrations. However, this action is weak at the so-called therapeutic concentrations achieved, and it is a non-selective inhibitor of phosphodiesterases. Other mechanisms may involve antagonism of adenosine receptors or increased secretion of adrenaline. In addition to its bronchodilator effect, which is weaker than that of inhaled β_2-agonists, theophylline may have act by inhibiting the activation of inflammatory cells such as T cells and macrophages, and by inhibiting airway microvascular leakage. Theophylline inhibits the late-phase response to allergen and the influx of eosinophils induced by allergen, and decreases the number of activated T cells in the airway mucosa.

Pharmacokinetics

Theophylline is readily absorbed from the gastrointestinal tract, and there are interindividual variations in clearance due to hepatic metabolism by cytochrome microsomal enzymes. Its plasma levels can be affected by many factors. For example, there may be increased clearance through enzymatic induction by drugs such as rifampicin, by smoking and a high-protein diet. Decreased clearance may occur in congestive cardiac failure, liver disease, old age and as a result of enzyme inhibition by many drugs, including cimetidine, erythromycin, ciprofloxacin and allopurinol. Many different slow-release formulations of theophylline or aminophylline are available for twice-daily administration or, also, once-daily administration. In order to achieve bronchodilator effects, a plasma concentration of 10–20 mg/L should be aimed for, although lower plasma concentrations may be associated with an 'anti-inflammatory' effect.

Clinical use

Theophylline may be used as a bronchodilator in the treatment of acute exacerbations of asthma. However, β_2-agonists remain the drug of choice, and theophylline should be used as second-line treatment when β_2-agonists have failed.

Theophylline, when used to achieve plasma concentrations of 10–20 mg/L, has a bronchodilator effect in patients with asthma, although its effect is less effective than inhaled β_2-agonists. It may have additive effects to that of inhaled β_2-agonists, and therefore may be used as an additional bronchodilator to short-acting inhaled β_2-agonists. Slow-release theophylline preparations may be particularly effective in patients with nocturnal asthma, although long-acting β-agonists may provide similar or better benefit. Addition of a low-dose theophylline, achieving therapeutic plasma concentrations of 8–15 mg/L, is as effective as doubling the dose of inhaled corticosteroids in patients not controlled by low or moderate doses of inhaled corticosteroids (Figure 5.11). Therefore, theophylline could be added to inhaled steroid therapy to improve asthma control.

Figure 5.11
The effect of adding low-dose theophylline to a medium-dose budesonide (400 μg twice daily) on change in FEV$_1$, compared to high-dose budesonide only (800 μg twice daily). Overall, the addition of theophylline provided a better effect than the high-dose budesonide alone. (Reproduced with permission from Evans (1997) *N. Engl. J. Med.* **337**, 1412–18. Copyright © 1997 Massachusetts Medical Society.)

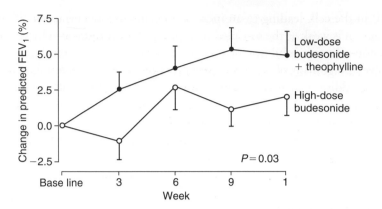

Side-effects

Serious side-effects, such as cardiac arrythmias and epileptic fits, may occur when plasma concentrations exceed 20 mg/L. However, other side-effects, such as nausea and vomiting, headaches, gastric discomfort such as acid reflux, diuresis and certain behavioural disturbances, may occur even at low plasma concentrations, although their incidence increases at higher plasma concentrations. These side-effects may be avoided by a more gradual build-up of plasma concentrations. Since beneficial 'anti-inflammatory' effects may be obtained at so-called subtherapeutic concentrations, low-dose theophylline may be used with avoidance of side-effects.

ANTICHOLINERGICS

Anticholinergics are specific antagonists of muscarinic receptors and inhibit bronchoconstriction induced by stimulation of cholinergic nerves. Therefore, anticholinergic drugs can protect against bronchoconstrictor stimuli such as sulphur dioxide, dusts, cold air, while being less effective against allergen challenge and exercise. They have no effect on mast-cell activation, microvascular leakage and inflammatory cells. Clinically, they are less effective bronchodilators and bronchoprotectors than β-agonists, although they are more effective in older patients with asthma. Nebulized anticholinergic drugs are effective in reversing bronchoconstriction in acute severe asthma. Although less effective than β-agonists, their effect is additive to those of nebulized β-agonists.

The available anticholinergic drugs are ipratropium bromide and oxitropium bromide, which cause a maximum degree of bronchodilatation by 30–60 min after inhalation, an effect persisting for ~6 hours. Tiotropium bromide, with a duration of effect of more than 36 hours, is a newly developed anticholinergic which will become available soon. Ipratropium bromide, available as a metered-dose inhaler and a nebulized preparation, is the most widely used. It may be used in elderly asthmatics in conjunction with a short-acting inhaled β-agonist four times daily. The greatest use for ipratropium bromide is in the treatment of acute severe asthma, when it is nebulized together with a β-agonist.

Because of little systemic absorption, there are very few systemic side-effects with inhaled ipratropium bromide. These include dryness of mouth, blurred vision and urinary retention. Ipratropium bromide has no significant effect in reducing mucus secretion or mucociliary clearance. However, it may precipitate glaucoma in elderly patients if nebulized to the face; hence, it is recommended that nebulization be given via a mouth piece rather than via a face mask. Ipratropium has a bitter taste. Paradoxical bronchoconstriction has been described previously with nebulized ipratropium bromide, perhaps due to hypotonicity and additives in the nebulized solution. This is less of a problem now.

Other treatments

ANTIHISTAMINES

Antihistamines have no place in the treatment of asthma. However, allergic problems that sometimes accompany asthma, such as allergic rhinitis, conjunctivitis and urticaria, should be treated with non-sedating antihistamines. Some patients with seasonal exacerbations of asthma and rhinitis find that antihistamines control their symptoms during the season. Ketotifen is an antihistamine, and claims have been made that it can prevent the onset of asthma. There is little evidence that it is effective in the treatment of asthma or that it can prevent the development of asthma.

IMMUNOTHERAPY

Specific allergen immunotherapy (desensitization, hyposensitization) is a technique by which IgE-mediated disease is treated with increasing doses of allergen, with the aim of decreasing sensitivity to that allergen. It is very effective for preventing life-threatening anaphylactic allergic reactions after stings by Hymenoptera (bees or wasps). Grass pollen immunotherapy is effective in grass-pollen-sensitive patients with severe hayfever symptoms unresponsive to usual pharmacological treatments. Long-term benefits are conferred for at least 3 years after stopping immunotherapy, and wheezing during the grass-pollen season is also controlled. A meta-analysis of 20 double-blind controlled studies showed a small, but significant, improvement in the control of asthma with immunotherapy to house dust mite and other allergens, in both adults and children. This analysis concluded that immunotherapy is a treatment option in highly selected patients with allergic asthma.

However, the use of immunotherapy in the treatment of asthma remains controversial, and comparative efficacy with other treatments, such as inhaled corticosteroid therapy, is not available. It is widely practised for the treatment of various allergic conditions, such as allergic rhinitis and asthma, in many European countries and in the USA. Following a report by the Committee of Safety of Medicines in 1986, recommending the need for accessible resuscitative measures when practising immunotherapy, it has rarely been used since. In the UK, immunotherapy is confined to monoallergic grass-pollen-sensitive patients and is administered in specialist allergy centres. Immunotherapy is not recommended in the British Thoracic Society's guidelines.

It is likely that with refinements in allergen derivatives by genetic engineering or synthetic peptide chemistry, or with the development of allergen-derived T-cell peptide epitopes, immunotherapy may be more effective and safer.

IMMUNOSUPPRESSIVE THERAPY AS STEROID-SPARING AGENTS

In controlled trials of patients needing oral corticosteroid therapy to control asthma, a number of immunosuppressive drugs, such as methotrexate, cyclosporin A and gold salts, have been shown to have some steroid-sparing effect. However, these drugs are associated with the development of potentially serious side-effects, and in clinical practice have not proven to be very useful. Occasional patients with severe asthma may still benefit from these therapies, which are best administered under close supervision in specialist asthma clinics.

ALTERNATIVE THERAPIES

Many patients with asthma seek alternative therapies such as acupuncture, homeopathy and herbal medicines. The spectrum of therapies ranges from herbal medicines, hypnosis, ionizer therapy, homeopathy, yoga and spinal manipulation. Some currently used therapies have been derived from herbal treatments, such as ephedrine from *Ma-huang*, anti-cholinergic alkaloids from *Datura stromanium*, theophylline from coffee and khellin (or sodium cromoglycate) from *Ammi visnaga*. A recent review of herbal medicines used for asthma examined the use of Chinese and Indian herbal medicines in 17 randomized clinical trials, and concluded that nine of these showed clinically relevant improvement in lung function and/or symptoms. But double-blind randomized studies were recommended. It is also important to note that some herbal medicines may be associated with severe toxic effects, that may occasionally be fatal. Acupuncture has some limited efficacy in reversing exercise-induced bronchonstriction, but its role in management of asthma is unclear.

There is no evidence of any anti-asthmatic effect of homeopathy or spinal manipulation. Yoga and hypnosis may be useful in the tense, anxious asthmatic patient. Objective improvement in peak flow and subjective improvement in symptoms score have been observed with yoga. The '*Buteyko*' technique of controlled breathing exercises has not been shown to lead to better control of asthma. Overall, the small benefits that may be derived from these therapies may evolve from a 'holistic' approach to asthma, which may be lacking in the physician's approach. More scientifically based trials are needed. When a patient seeks alternative treatments, the physician needs to safeguard him or her against quacks and other forms of unregulated over-the-counter therapies, and must ascertain that the patient's asthma is being managed as best as possible with conventional methods and therapies.

Inhaler devices

GENERAL CONSIDERATIONS

Many treatments for asthma are delivered directly to the airways in the form of aerosols or small particles, for rapid onset of action (e.g. β-agonists) or for minimizing side-effects (e.g. corticosteroids). However, not all asthma drugs work when delivered directly to the airways (e.g. leukotriene inhibitors). Since the mainstay of asthma treatments are delivered directly to the airways, it is important to be aware of the different types of delivery devices available. An ideal inhaler device delivers a predetermined dose of drugs to the lungs, via an easy to use and reproducible inhaler, usually with minimal deposition at other sites. A plethora of different devices is now available on the market (Figure 5.12), since each pharmaceutical company uses a different device with their products. Thus, patients and doctors have a wide range of devices to choose from. Drug delivery to the lungs depends on factors arising from both the patient and from the device.

Patient factors

Many patients may find it difficult to coordinate actuation and inspiration precisely with a metered dose inhaler, or to inhale forcefully enough to use a dry-powder inhaler, or they may find the device too 'complicated' to use. Therefore, it is important to choose the correct device that the patient will find easy to use and will use correctly. Once taught, the inhaler technique needs to be checked constantly, and any difficulties identified and corrected, or else another more suitable device is offered. Adherence to treatment may also influenced by the choice of inhaler device. When asthma is poorly controlled despite the prescription of appropriate treatments, inhaler techniques and adherence to treatment should be checked and remedied, if necessary.

Figure 5.12
Examples of inhaler devices and holding chambers (spacers) available. The inhaler devices shown are: pressurized metered-dose inhaler, an Autohaler®, a Turbohaler®, an Accuhaler®, and a Diskhaler®. The holding chambers shown are: Volumatic®, Nebuhaler® and Aerochamber®.

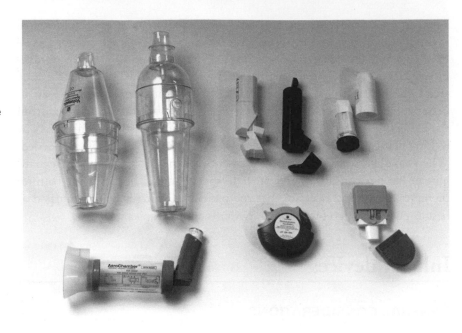

Box 5.4
Inhalers

Metered-dose inhaler

1. Advantages:
   (a) small and portable;
   (b) usually cheap;
   (c) rapid to use.

2. Disadvantages:
   (a) good coordination is essential;
   (b) children less than 6 years of age cannot use;
   (c) elderly patients, those with arthritis or with coordination problems cannot use.

Dry-powder inhaler

1. Advantages:
   (a) small and portable;
   (b) coordination between priming and inspiration is not important;
   (c) can be used by children from 5–6 years.

2. Disadvantages:
   (a) need rapid inspiration;
   (b) generally more expensive;
   (c) not suitable for children below 5 years of age.

Inhaler factors

Deposition of particles in the airways is optimal with particle sizes of 1–3 μm diameter, and most therapeutic aerosols are within a particle size of 1–5 μm diameter. Particles equal to or greater than 10 μm deposit in the mouth and throat, and do not penetrate into the airways because of the sudden change in airflow in the upper airway, and because of the cough it induces. Each inhaler has its own characteristics that will determine the amount of respirable to non-respirable particles, and the extent or pattern of delivery to the airways will depend on the coordination, on the inspiratory flow characteristics and also on the presence of airflow obstruction. There are three types of dispersal of a medication into an aerosol for inhalation: pressurized metered-dose inhaler, dry-powder inhaler (Box 5.4) or nebulization.

PRESSURIZED METERED-DOSE INHALER

The pressurized metered-dose inhaler (pMDI) was the first effective inhaler device to be developed, and is the most popular form of inhaler device in many countries, including the UK. The medication is mixed with a propellant in a reservoir and released through a metering device when it is activated. The propellant helps to propel and disaggregate the particles. One spray is released with each activation into the mouth, from where it is inhaled. The propellant has usually been a chlorofluorocarbon (CFC), but because CFCs damage the Earth's ozone layer, they will be gradually replaced by hydrofluorocarbons. The pMDI can be manually or breath actuated.

Manually actuated pMDIs

The manually actuated pMDI is convenient, quick to actuate and usually relatively inexpensive. The technique consists of shaking the device, then placing the mouthpiece of the pMDI in the mouth, activating the canister, while at the same time taking an inspiratory manoeuvre to total lung capacity, then holding the breath for usually 10 seconds. This complex manoeuvre, which requires good coordination and psychomotor skills to ensure that the correct sequence of events is performed, needs to be taught and checked regularly, and is difficult for young and older patients and for physically impaired adults. Up to 30 per cent of adult patients have been reported to have an inadequate technique, but this is likely to be higher. The most common mistakes include not shaking the canister, inhaling too rapidly, not coordination between actuation and inspiration, and not holding the breath long enough. Some patients may stop inhaling when they feel the particles hitting the back of their throat. The amount of drug delivered to the lower respiratory tract varies from 7 to 20 per cent, very much dependent on the patient's inhaler technique, and more than 80 per cent deposits in the throat and oropharynx.

Breath-actuated pMDIs

Breath-actuated pMDIs are triggered during inhalation, usually at flow rate of around 30 L/min, which reduces the need for coordination of actuation of canister and inspiration. These are particularly useful for elderly and for handicapped patients, and are particularly advantageous compared to the conventional pMDI. Their use in very young children is not clear, and it is recommended that they are used in older children and adults. There is no advantage of the breath-actuated inhaler over the conventional pMDI in patients who are already using conventional pMDI with a good technique. Breath-actuated pMDIs are bulkier and less portable than conventional pMDIs.

Spacer devices

Two main types of spacer devices exist: extension devices and holding chambers. These devices reduce oropharyngeal deposition and improve lower respiratory tract deposition. Both types of spacer devices increase the distance between the source point of aerosolized drug and the upper airway such that the propellant can evaporate, leading to a reduction in particle size of the aerosol droplets, together with trapping of the larger non-respirable particles. With the extension tube, however, the patient still needs to be able to coordinate actuation with inspiration.

Holding chambers provide a reservoir of drug which is provided from the MDI, and the patient breathes from the chamber. They reduce the need for coordination between actuation and inhalation, since the drug particles are trapped within the holding chamber. They are generally easier for children and older patients to use than a pMDI alone. Chambers that contain a valve allow for tidal breathing from the reservoir, particularly useful in children. Face masks attached to holding chambers are now used for treating very young children.

Usually, drugs are administered as single actuations into a spacer, and inhaled immediately afterwards with a single deep inspiration. Alternatively, a series of smaller breaths appears to be as effective. This should be repeated until all the prescribed dose is taken (usually two puffs). It is not advisable to use multiple actuations into the spacer. The use of a large-volume spacer reduces oropharyngeal deposition, and lowers the incidence of local side-effects, such as oropharyngeal candidiasis, and absorption from the oropharynx and gastrointestinal tract. It is advisable to wash the spacer device monthly with washing-up liquid and to allow it to dry, in order to remove static charges on the plastic and polycarbonate walls of the spacer that reduce the output of particles from the spacer.

CFC-free MDIs

Currently, many manufacturers are phasing out their CFC-containing MDIs, to be replaced by CFC-free MDIs. New MDIs therefore have to be redesigned to ensure compatibility with new propellants. CFC-free formulations of salbutamol and of beclomethasone are now licensed in the UK. There are differences between CFC-containing and CFC-free MDIs, even for the same drug. A new HFC-salbutamol MDI produces the same particle size and dose as a CFC-containing Ventolin® MDI, but not when used with a spacer device. A HFC-beclomethasone MDI, Qvar®, releases smaller particle sizes than a CFC-containing beclomethasone, with a higher deposition in the lung periphery, and control of asthma appears to be obtained with half the dose of Qvar® as BDP from a conventional MDI. Therefore, it is necessary to specify on prescription the exact brand needed, whether CFC-free or containing, the exact doses to be taken and the specific type of spacer device needed. With time, a full range of CFC-free MDIs will become available, and CFC-containing MDIs will be removed from the market. The changeover should be carefully managed, and good communication between health professionals and patients is necessary for a successful transition.

DRY-POWDER INHALER

Dry-powder inhalers (DPIs) deliver either the pure drug or drug mixed with a suitable inert compound, often lactose, and do not require propellants. They are activated by inspiratory effort, and therefore there is no need for coordinating firing with inhalation. When first developed, single doses of drug were contained in a capsule, but later designs have incorporated multiple doses. These are available either as single doses from individual capsules inserted into the device (Spinhaler®, Rotahaler®) or from a blister pack or metered dose of powder (Diskhaler®, Accuhaler®, Turbohaler®). The deposition of the powder depends very much on the inspiratory flow rates. Devices will differ according to how inspiratory flow rates affect particle size, how the drug is stored and the dose metered, and the presence of dose counters or warnings of empty device. DPIs are not suitable for children under 6 years old, because they are usually unable to generate inspiratory flow of 30 L/min. However, use of DPIs does not involve coordination between inspiration and actuation, and they are therefore an alternative for those who have trouble using a conventional pMDI. Oropharyngeal deposition remains high and patients should be advised to rinse the mouth and throat with water after inhaling from a DPI in order to reduce local side-effects and absorption.

Diskhaler® and Accuhaler®

The Diskhaler® is a multidose DPI for delivering salbutamol, salmeterol, BDP or fluticasone. Four or eight pre-metered doses mixed with lactose are sealed in individual foil blisters. The Accuhaler® device contains 60 doses in blisters on a foil strip, and has a dose counter that locks when the device is empty. It is used to deliver salbutamol, salmeterol, fluticasone, or the combination of salmeterol and fluticasone. It has been designed to deliver a similar dose to that received from a correctly used MDI without a spacer. At inspiratory flow rates of 30–90 L/min, a respirable fraction of 16–21 per cent is obtained.

Turbohaler®

The Turbohaler® delivers turbutaline, formoterol or budesonide, and the combination of formoterol and budesonide. It has a powder reservoir for 50, 100 or 200 individual doses, which is dispensed by a volumetric metering system. It needs to be primed by holding it upright and twisting the base. The pure drug is delivered without any carrier admixture and is tasteless. The device should be stored in a dry place. Patients should be told to inhale forcefully and deeply. At an adult average inspiratory flow of 60 L/min, lung deposition is twice that of the same dose inhaled correctly from a pMDI. The dose reaching the lungs drops by 50 per cent when the inspiratory flow rate falls to 30–40 L/min. Control of asthma in 5–15-year-old children was achieved with half the dose of budesonide when administered from a Turbohaler® compared to a pMDI with spacer.

NEBULIZERS

The most common nebulizers are jet nebulizers, in which a jet of air from a compressor entrains some of the liquid drug from the reservoir and breaks it into fine particles as it hits a baffle. The particles are inhaled by the patient, either from an open mask or from a mouthpiece. An ultrasonic nebulizer uses a piezoelectric crystal which vibrates on passage of an electric current, to produce a spray above the liquid contained in a reservoir. Jet nebulizers are cheaper and more robust than ultrasonic nebulizers. They do not rely on the patient's cooperation or coordination. More drug is delivered to the lungs when inhaled from a mouthpiece than from a face mask, and during quiet breathing compared to rapid breathing. The main indication for using a nebulizer is in the treatment of acute severe asthma in adults and children, or in ill patients who cannot use an MDI or PDI, and need urgent bronchodilator therapy, or in severely obstructed patients. Nebulizers vary greatly in their outputs and an efficient nebulizer should deliver about 50 per cent of particles below 5 μm diameter over 5–15-min periods. Usually less than 10 per cent of the dose gets into the lungs.

A new generation of nebulizers with greater efficiency and more respirable particle generation are becoming increasingly available, such as open-vent nebulizers, breath-enhanced open-vent nebulizers, and intelligent dosimetric nebulizers. These have special features that increase nebulizer outputs, and shorten nebulization times.

Management of chronic asthma and acute severe asthma

6

Introduction

One of the most important advances over the past 15 years in asthma management in the UK has been the setting up of consensus national approaches to the management of asthma by a team of experts, composed of hospital adult physicians, paediatricians and primary-care physicians. This arose in the 1980s because of particular concern raised by hospital-based physicians interested in the treatment of asthma, regarding the increasing problem of asthma and the inadequate assessment and intervention that was being undertaken at both primary- and secondary-care levels. This led to the setting up of 'guidelines' in many countries, specifically aimed at the management of asthma, both acute (short-term) and chronic (long-term) asthma, in adults as well as in children. The first of many guidelines appeared in 1989–90 for adults, and for children. Since then, other guidelines have appeared, usually put together by groups of expert physicians in their respective countries. The asthma guidelines in the UK were produced under the auspices of the British Thoracic Society and published in 1990. The US National Heart, Lung and Blood Institute, together with the World Health Organization, has produced the Global Initiative for Asthma Management and Prevention (GINA). The guidelines are a useful starting point for increasing awareness of the problem of asthma, setting up standards, for use as a basis for audit and for education of physicians and patients about best practice of managing asthma. Overall, the main objective of having guidelines is to decrease the morbidity and mortality associated with this chronic disease. The guidelines represent a consensus amongst expert physicians in the field of asthma, and many of the aspects of guidelines, particularly specific interventions in specific groups of asthmatics, may not be based on evidence backed by randomized placebo-controlled trials, but often on best clinical practice. In areas where insufficient data exist, common sense and experience are applied until more definite evidence is obtained. Thus, the guidelines offer a framework for the best clinical practice at the time. Guidelines may therefore be modified with time, and already some guidelines have been revised in the light of new evidence and with the arrival of novel treatment modalities. Increasingly, future guidelines will take the approach of evidence-based medicine and will provide the level of evidence there is to support specific interventions or treatments in asthma.

Who cares for the asthmatic patient?

The care of asthmatics occurs at several levels of medical care and also in the home and work environment, since asthma is a chronic condition that affects most age groups, and that may present at any time and at different levels of severity. Asthma continues, and will continue, to be managed mainly at primary-care level, where it accounts for a substantial proportion of the workload of the general practitioner. There was a twofold increase in the number of patient consultations for asthma in 1991–92, compared to the previous 10 years. Asthma care in general practice consists of diagnosis, delivery and supervision of care, and treatment of acute asthma attacks. With such a wide and large remit, the organization of the general practice needs to be supported adequately, and trained asthma nurses have become important members of the general practice team. The setting-up of asthma clinics in general practice, generally run by asthma nurses, has been seen as relatively successful in improving the supervision of asthma care, particularly in improving compliance to treatment, the use of inhalers and in implementation of self-management plans. In the management of acute asthma episodes, the severity of the attack should be assessed, followed by provision of initial treatment. Follow-up of patients who present with an acute attack is of prime importance, because these episodes usually indicate poorly controlled asthma and can be prevented.

Within the community, the school is an important place because the prevalence of asthma is particularly high amongst children. Supervision of chronic asthma care could take place here, and episodes of asthma can occur and reliever medication may be needed in school (for example, after exercise, or delivery of routine preventive therapy). The role of the school nurse is important in this respect, and some commitment of the teaching staff is needed. The role of the teacher or of a designated teacher (in the absence of a school nurse) in supervision of asthma during school hours remains to be defined.

In secondary care, patients with more severe asthma are usually followed, having been referred from primary care or from the emergency department where the patient has been treated or admitted for a severe attack of asthma. An important proportion of such patients fail to attend follow-up, and it is in this area that a primary–secondary care coordinated approach may be most beneficial. Within the hospital, the components of the service will include the emergency department, the medical ward, the intensive care unit and the asthma clinic, with the physicians (including geriatricians), paediatricians and the asthma nurse forming the asthma management team. Other personnel who may be included are: physiotherapist, clinical psychologist, dietitian, pharmacist and social worker. Often, the handover of care from the paediatrician to the adult physician of the teenage/adolescent asthmatic has to be handled carefully. The hospital approach to management must be multidisciplinary, and implement strategies to reduce morbidity by providing education and self-management skills to patients.

Asthma is a chronic disease that needs regular follow-up, as much for assessing the disease as for ensuring that treatment is being complied with and that side-effects of drugs are recognized. Continuing care is necessary for those with persistent symptoms, in spite of significant amount of medication, and monthly or 2-monthly visits may be necessary. These patients should also be seen in a specialist asthma clinic. Patients who are controlled adequately on asthma medication should also be reviewed regularly at 3–4-monthly intervals. At each review, the degree of asthma symptoms is reviewed together with lung function, and self-recording of peak flow charts examined, treatment is adjusted as necessary, the self-management plan reviewed, drugs prescribed, inhalation techniques checked and aspects of education reinforced.

Overall plan and aims of management

The principles of asthma management are set out in Box 6.1. The important components are:

1. The criteria for control of asthma are identified and set as standards of care that aim at asthma symptom prevention with the achievement of a normal lifestyle and lung function (Box 6.2). Control of asthma should be accompanied by a minimum of side-effects from therapy.
2. Although preventive measures (e.g. allergen avoidance) are important to set in place, the mainstay of treatment of asthma remains to a large extent pharmacological. The aim of therapy should be to treat the underlying cause of asthma, which is inflammatory, rather than depend on medication that relieves symptoms, such as bronchodilators. An anti-inflammatory approach should therefore be the primary treatment to control asthma.
3. A stepwise approach to therapy is recommended. Therapy may start with low doses and progressively increased in scale, or may be initiated at the 'right' level for the level of severity. Many patients may benefit by having their asthma brought rapidly under control by high doses of inhaled corticosteroids before reducing therapy to reach the minimum dose consistent with achieving and sustaining control.

Cure, defined as the absence of symptoms and airflow obstruction after stopping treatment for a period of time, is not currently available for asthma, and the main objectives of the treatment are to control the disease and to

Box 6.1
Principles of asthma management

1. To diagnose and evaluate asthma severity and establish criteria to be achieved to control asthma.
2. To advise about avoidance of triggers and preventive measures, such as allergen avoidance.
3. To establish pharmacological therapy. A stepwise approach to therapy is recommended.
4. To educate about asthma, instruct about drug administration, and propose self-management plans for the patient.
5. To set up follow-up measures for the patient.

Box 6.2
Goals of asthma management

1. Achieve and maintain control of symptoms.
2. Prevent asthma exacerbation.
3. Maintain pulmonary function as close to normal levels as possible.
4. Maintain normal activity levels, including exercise.
5. Avoid adverse effects from asthma medications.
6. Prevent development of irreversible airway obstruction.
7. Prevent asthma mortality.

prevent irreversible airway damage. Control of asthma is defined as absence of symptoms and exacerbations, no need for rescue medication, normal levels of activity including exercise and sports, normal lung function and minimal adverse effects from medication. In many patients, control of asthma can be achieved using currently available treatment. Because asthma is episodic, the amount of control can also be assessed by the number of symptom-free days or nights, or by the use of reliever medication. In some patients, complete control cannot be achieved, particularly in patients with severe asthma, in those not compliant with, or unwilling to take, medication, or in those in whom the risk of side-effects from medication is too high.

Attaining normal lung function may be impossible in asthma due to the presence of irreversible changes in the airways. Usually, a normal lung function, measured in terms of the predicted normal range for FEV_1 or PEFR, is taken as being more than 80 per cent. In patients with some irreversible damage, the personal best PEF or FEV_1 from historical records may be used as the reference value. There is still lack of clarity regarding the necessity for, and ability to achieve, normal lung function, but the consensus is that this should be an important goal. Indirect evidence suggests that the risk of irreversible obstruction increases with suboptimal or delayed treatment of asthma. There is increasing evidence that patients with asthma have a faster decline in FEV_1 over time than non-asthmatics. Early treatment of asthma could prevent this irreversible airflow limitation. Bronchial responsiveness has not been recommended as a measure for normalization.

A reduction in mortality is another important goal of asthma management, since many asthma deaths are considered avoidable by appropriate management. The recent fall in asthma mortality in the UK may have resulted from improvement in asthma management ensuing from dissemination of guidelines. There is very little information on the effects of treatments on asthma mortality, and a recent epidemiological study indicated that inhaled corticosteroid therapy could reduce asthma deaths.

Avoidance of causes, triggers and worsening factors of asthma

Although much of asthma management is pharmacologically based, special attention should be given to the avoidance of exposure to factors that worsen asthma. This should be tailored to each patient's needs, since the type of triggers that cause worsening of asthma varies from patient to patient. These potential triggers are discussed in Chapter 4. Avoidance measures need to be adapted to the patient's allergies, lifestyle and severity of asthma.

Exposure to cold air and exercise are part of everyday life, and could be prevented with good preventive treatment of asthma. Use of a β-agonist aerosol, or sodium cromoglycate or nedocromil sodium, prior to such exposures can minimize these attacks. Avoiding passive or active smoking is important since these increase the frequency and severity of symptoms of asthmatic patients. Exposure to cigarette smoke can reduce the effectiveness of asthma medication. It is mandatory for patients with asthma not to smoke, to give up smoking and to reduce exposure to cigarette smoke. Both indoor and outdoor pollutants can worsen asthma symptoms or provoke acute episodes. Indoor pollution from heating and cooking systems can be prevented by adequate ventilation of furnaces/fires. Outdoor pollution may be more difficult to avoid, and on days of significant levels of pollutants such as sulphur dioxide, nitric oxide and ozone, it is advisable to stay indoors, and increase asthma medication as necessary. It is, however, more difficult to avoid small particulate pollutants (PM_{10}), and a general approach to curb the source of these pollutants from car exhaust fumes would be more effective. Medications such as β-adrenergic blockers or muscarinic agonists should be avoided in patients with asthma. Other medications such as aspirin or non-steroidal anti-inflammatory drugs such as indomethacin, flurbiprofen, ibuprofen and diclofenac may provoke asthma attacks in a subgroup of asthmatics, usually with a severe form of asthma combined with rhinosinusitis. These subjects should therefore avoid these drugs. Rarely, some asthmatics experience attacks with ingestion of sulphite-containing foods or drinks, particularly wine.

COMORBIDITY FACTORS

Certain associated conditions, such as rhinosinusitis and gastro-oesophageal reflux, may aggravate asthma. These should be treated appropriately.

AEROALLERGENS

Avoidance of house dust mite and companion animals, particularly cats, has the greatest potential for benefit, and may be important, beginning at or even before birth. Clinical trials using measures to reduce house dust mites in the homes of children and adults have shown benefits in terms of asthma control, but reducing exposure to low levels is not easy. In many studies, significant reductions in house dust mite allergen levels were not achieved in the home. The greatest benefits that have been observed relate to asthmatic children, sensitive to house dust mites, who were removed from their homes to high-altitude alpine areas for periods of up to 9 months. This led to improvement in bronchial responsiveness and measures of inflammation. House dust mites thrive in high humidity, and decreasing indoor humidity to less than 50 per cent is associated with lower house dust mite concentrations. Encasing mattresses in a vapour-impermeable barrier is effective in decreasing exposure to house dust mites, as is laundering bed linens in hot water (60°C). Removal of carpets is most effective, but use of acaricides or liquid nitrogen to freeze carpeting can also lead to short-term reductions in house dust mite concentrations. While general advice about some of these measures needs to be given and enforced as much as possible, it would ideally be best to measure the level of house dust mite in the home in order to measure the efficacy of the avoidance measures. This is not generally possible.

Removal of pets from the home is the most effective means of reducing cat or dog allergen. However, in practice, this is not easily done, for various psychosocial reasons. Cat allergens may persist for up to 6 months in the house following the animal's removal. Weekly washing of the cat may reduce allergen exposure, but it is not easy to wash a cat! Cat allergens may be found in schools and hospitals, associated with upholstered furniture and textile floor coverings, having been spread by visitors.

Pharmacological management

The individual drugs used to treat asthma have been discussed in Chapter 5. A short version of the stepwise approach for pharmacological management is

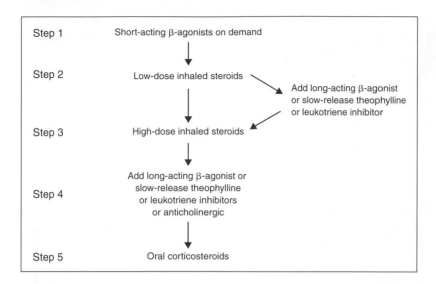

Figure 6.1
Pharmacological treatment of asthma using a stepwise approach.

shown in Figure 6.1, with a longer version in Figure 6.2. Although five steps of treatment are shown, i.e. those included in the British guidelines, other guidelines use only four steps, with the steps 4 and 5 of the British guidelines combined into a single step representing severe asthmatics.

STEP 1, FOR MILD ASTHMA WITH NORMAL LUNG FUNCTION: INHALED β_2-AGONISTS, AS REQUIRED, FOR LESS THAN ONCE DAILY

- Use inhaled short-acting β-agonists (usually 1–2 puffs) as required for symptom relief. For children, the inhaled route is more effective and much preferred than oral preparations.
- Ensure that patients have a good inhaler technique.
- If inhaled β-agonists are needed more than three times per week, move to Step 2.

STEP 2, FOR MILD TO MODERATE ASTHMA: REGULAR INHALED ANTI-INFLAMMATORY DRUG

- Add a regular anti-inflammatory agent (preventer/prophylactic).
- Continue to use a short-acting inhaled β-agonist as reliever medication.
- Low-dose inhaled corticosteroid (400–600 μg beclomethasone or budesonide, 200–400 μg fluticasone) is the treatment of choice.
- In children, a trial of sodium cromoglycate or nedocromil sodium may be given and, if not effective, changed to corticosteroid. Most paediatricians consider inhaled corticosteroids to be the first treatment of choice at this step.
- A leukotriene inhibitor is an alternative.

Prescribe a peak flow meter and monitor response to treatment

Notes
- Patients should start treatment at the step most appropriate to the initial severity. A rescue course of prednisolone may be needed at any time and at any step. The aim is to achieve early control of the condition and then to reduce treatment.
- Until growth is complete any child requiring beclomethasone or budesonide >800 µg daily or fluticasone >500 µg daily should be referred to a paediatrician with an interest in asthma.

- Avoidance of provoking factors where possible
- Patient's involvement and education
- Selection of best inhaler device
- Treatment stepped up as necessary to achieve good control
- Treatment stepped down if control of asthma good

Stepping down:

Review treatment every three to six months. If control is achieved, a stepwise reduction in treatment may be possible. In patients whose treatment was recently started at step 4 or 5 or included steroid tablets for gaining control of asthma this reduction may take place after a short interval. In other patients with chronic asthma a three to six month period of stability should be shown before slow stepwise reduction is undertaken

Step 5:

Addition of regular steroid tablets

Inhaled short-acting β-agonists as required with inhaled beclomethasone or budesonide 800–2000 µg daily or fluticasone 400–1000 µg daily via a large-volume spacer and one or more of the long-acting bronchodilators
plus
regular prednisolone tablets in a single daily dose

Step 4:

High-dose inhaled steroids and regular bronchodilators

Inhaled short-acting β-agonists as required with inhaled beclomethasone or budesonide 800–2000 µg daily or fluticasone 400–1000 µg daily via a large-volume spacer
plus
a sequential therapeutic trial of one or more of:
- inhaled long-acting β-agonists
- sustained-release theophylline
- inhaled ipratropium or oxitropium
- long-acting β-agonist tablets
- high-dose inhaled bronchodilators
- cromoglycate or nedocromil

Step 3:

High-dose inhaled steroids or low-dose inhaled steroids plus long-acting inhaled β-agonist bronchodilator

Inhaled short-acting β-agonists as required
plus either
beclomethasone or budesonide increased to 800–2000 µg daily or fluticasone 400–1000 µg daily via a large-volume spacer
or
beclomethasone or budesonide 100–400 µg twice daily plus salmeterol 50 µg twice daily. In a very small number of patients who experience side-effects with high-dose inhaled steroids, either the long-acting inhaled β-agonist option is used or a sustained release theophylline may be added to step 2 medication. Cromoglycate or nedocromil may also be tried

Step 2:

Regular inhaled anti-inflammatory agents

Inhaled short-acting β-agonists as required
plus
beclomethasone or budesonide 100–400 µg twice-daily or fluticasone 50–200 µg twice daily. Alternatively, use cromoglycate or nedocromil sodium, but if control is not achieved start inhaled steroids

Step 1:

Occasional use of relief bronchodilators

Inhaled short-acting β-agonists 'as required' for symptom relief are acceptable. If they are needed more than once daily, move to step 2. Before altering a treatment step ensure that the patient is having the treatment and has a good inhaler technique. Address any fears

Outcome of steps 1–3: control of asthma
- Minimal (ideally no) chronic symptoms, including nocturnal symptoms
- Minimal (infrequent) exacerbations
- Minimal need for relieving bronchodilators
- No limitations on activities, including exercise
- Circadian variation in peak expiratory flow (PEF) <20%
- PEF ≥ 80% of predicted or best
- Minimal (or no) adverse effects from medicine

Outcome of steps 4–5: best possible results
- Least possible symptoms
- Least possible need for relieving bronchodilators
- Least possible limitation of activity
- Least possible variation in PEF
- Best PEF
- Least adverse effects from medicine

Figure 6.2

Management of chronic asthma in adults and schoolchildren according to the guidelines of the British Thoracic Society. (Reproduced with permission of the BMJ Publishing Group from the British Thoracic Society (1997) *Thorax* **52 (suppl. 1)**.)

STEP 3, FOR MODERATE TO SEVERE ASTHMA: HIGH-DOSE INHALED CORTICOSTEROIDS OR LOW-DOSE CORTICOSTEROID TOGETHER WITH REGULAR BRONCHODILATORS

- Use short-acting β-agonists as required for symptom relief.
- Increase inhaled corticosteroid to maximum doses for adults (2000 μg beclomethasone or 1600 μg budesonide or 1000 μg of fluticasone). In children, the usual maximal dose is approximately halved.
- Alternatively, add a regular twice-daily, inhaled, long-acting β-agonist (salmeterol or formoterol) to the lower dose of inhaled corticosteroid.
- Alternative medications that may be added at this step include a low dose of slow-release theophylline or leukotriene inhibitors.

STEP 4, FOR SEVERE ASTHMA: HIGH-DOSE INHALED CORTICOSTEROIDS TOGETHER WITH REGULAR BRONCHODILATORS

- Use short-acting β-agonist as required for symptom relief, and maximal inhaled corticosteroids, as for Step 3.
- Add a regular, twice-daily, long-acting β-agonist such as salmeterol or formoterol, or, alternatively, slow-release theophylline, or a leukotriene inhibitor.
- An inhaled anticholinergic such as ipratropium bromide may be combined with the β-agonist. It is not known whether additional benefits will derive from adding long-acting β-agonists with theophylline and/or leukotriene inhibitor.

STEP 5, FOR SEVERE ASTHMA UNRESPONSIVE AT STEP 4: REGULAR ORAL CORTICOSTEROIDS

- Use short-acting inhaled β-agonist as required for symptom relief.
- Inhaled corticosteroids at the maximum dose.
- Add a regular, twice-daily, long-acting β-agonist such as salmeterol or formoterol, or, alternatively, slow-release theophylline, or a leukotriene inhibitor.
- Add a regular oral corticosteroid (usually prednisolone) at the lowest dose that controls the symptoms. This should be given as a single dose in the morning. In children, alternate-day corticosteroid may be tried.
- A trial of nebulized inhaled steroids may be given, particularly in those with moderately severe airways obstruction.
- Steroid-sparing agents such as methotrexate and cyclosporin A may also be tried in those with high-dose oral steroid requirements.

Box 6.3
Definition of control of
asthma

1. Minimal chronic symptoms (ideally no symptoms), including nocturnal symptoms.
2. Minimal or infrequent exacerbation.
3. Minimal need for β_2-agonist used on demand, ideally none.
4. No limitations on activities, including exercise.
5. Peak expiratory flow circadian variation (<20 per cent).
6. (Near) normal peak expiratory flow rate.
7. Minimal or no adverse effects from medication.

STEP-DOWN: REDUCTION IN ASTHMA THERAPY ONCE CONTROL IS ACHIEVED AT A GIVEN STEP

Treatment should be reviewed every 2 months, and at each review it is important to determine whether the treatment should be re-adjusted. In patients in whom asthma is well controlled with symptom-free periods and little or no rescue bronchodilator use, a step-down in treatment should be considered. It is important that the treatment be tailored to the needs of the patients as much as possible, e.g. patients with seasonal asthma should have step-up treatments during the season. The criteria for control of asthma are shown in Box 6.3.

Education and self-management

Because asthma is a chronic, variable and lifelong disease, patients and their families must be prepared to make lifestyle changes and adhere to medication. They must also be able to make decisions about the severity of their symptoms, about the need to adjust their therapies to severity or the need to seek medical help. In a chronic disease such as asthma, it is important to involve the patient in decision-making for good management. Compliance to medication and adherence to the advice of the physician depend on the patient understanding of the nature of the disease as well as the benefits of self-management. Regular visits to the physician are important for ensuring good treatment outcomes. Asthma education is an essential component of the management of asthma, with the goal of asthma education being the control of asthma by improving knowledge and changing behaviour. A number of studies have examined the impact of asthma education and self-management on healthcare costs and patient well-being. A reduction in hospital admissions, in emergency room visits, in unscheduled visits to the doctor, days off work or school and nocturnal asthma, and short-lived improvements in feeling of well-being and cost-effectiveness have been shown, particularly in the more severely affected patients.

- Asthma as a long-term, treatable disease.
- Information about airway inflammation and how bronchospasm occurs.
- The rationale for the use of anti-inflammatory drugs and bronchodilators.
- Instruction on the use of an inhaler, and use of a peak flow meter for monitoring.
- Determining the signs and symptoms of deterioration.
- Steps to take when deterioration occurs.
- Setting up of an action plan and how to implement it.
- Avoidance of trigger factors.
- Take appropriate action to prevent and treat symptoms in different situations.
- Reasons for regular follow-up and regular medication.
- Identify potential problems relating to compliance.
- Use of medical resources for chronic and acute care.

Box 6.4
Contents of self-management educational programmes

Several strategies are available for asthma education, although none of these is entirely sufficient on its own. Certain principles appear to work: asthma education should not rely on written or videotaped material alone, is effective only in the presence of effective asthma therapy, and must be provided at each patient contact. The essential components of an educational programme for the asthmatic are as shown in Box 6.4.

The following points in the management programme are essential:

- Educate patients to develop a partnership in asthma management.
- Assess and monitor asthma severity with objective measures of lung function.
- Avoid or control asthma triggers.
- Establish medication plans for chronic management.
- Establish plans for managing exacerbations.
- Provide regular follow-up care.

PEFR HOME MONITORING

Utilization of the peak flow meter to assess severity of the disease has allowed the patient to gain more control over disease management. Not all patients need to monitor peak flow measurements (particularly not those with mild asthma), but those with more severe disease, those with an insidious deterioration of their asthma, those with a poor perception of deteriorating dyspnoea or those prone to exacerbations of asthma find this useful sometimes in taking pre-emptive action, such as increasing the level of asthma medication.

Box 6.5
Self-management plan:
an example

- Best PEFR: 500 L/min.
- Asthma under control: PEFR >85 per cent best (425 L/min): use regular treatment.
- Asthma getting worse: PEFR <85 per cent best (<425 L/min): double dose of inhaled steroids.
- Asthma severe: PEFR <70 per cent best (<350 L/min): start course of oral prednisolone.
- Asthma emergency: PEFR <50 per cent best (<250 L/min): go to hospital emergency immediately or call for ambulance.

PEFR monitoring has been advocated as useful in the detection of exacerbations of asthma. However, in many patients, symptoms are as sensitive as the peak flow in detecting deterioration. The warning signs of an impending asthma exacerbation are as follows: increasing dyspnoea, nocturnal wheeze, a combination of wheeze, cough and mucus secretion, increasing use of short-acting β-agonist and increased exercise-induced asthma. PEFR monitoring is particularly good in patients who have difficulty in recognizing these symptoms as worsening of their asthma, and in patients with very severe asthma, by helping them to determine whether symptoms are due to reduced airflow.

Home peak flow monitoring should be linked to an appropriate action plan. The personalized action plan is made possible by the use of the peak flow meter, when important signs of deterioration can be recognized by certain falls in the peak flow measurement and particular instructions are given to the patient for increasing treatments or getting immediate advice from the physician. Such an approach has been shown to lead to better control of asthma. Most plans advise a doubling of inhaled corticosteroids and/or adding a course of oral steroids, and contacting a physician when emergency therapy is indicated (Box 6.5). However, the benefit of doubling a dose of corticosteroids has not been documented precisely. On the basis of PEFR, decrease by a given percentage leads to specific recommendations, usually a reduction to 80 per cent of the best value is an indication for augmentation of regular treatment, and to 60–70 per cent for initiating a course of oral corticosteroids.

Asthma in pregnancy

Asthma is present in about 5 per cent of pregnant women and most frequently complicates pregnancy. The course of asthma during pregnancy may remain unchanged, improve or worsen, but overall asthma control tends to improve during the final month of pregnancy. Poorly controlled asthma may affect maternal safety and pregnancy outcome for both mother and child. Treated asthmatic pregnant women have less adverse infant and maternal outcomes than those who are less-well treated. Therefore, it is important to control asthma during pregnancy. Use of the most common drugs for asthma (β_2-agonists, theophylline, sodium cromoglycate, inhaled corticosteroids) have not been shown to be associated with increased perinatal risks and congenital malformations. Oral corticosteroids, particularly if used over long periods, have been associated with an increased risk of pre-eclampsia, ante- or post-partum haemorrhage, low birth weight, preterm birth and hyperbilirubinaemia.

In managing the asthmatic pregnant patient, the physician should discuss with the patient the consequences for both mother and baby of uncontrolled asthma, and the importance of controlling asthma with available drugs. Treatment should take the same stepped approach as in the non-pregnant patient, using the same drugs, particularly inhaled corticosteroids, short- and long-acting β-agonists, theophylline and systemic corticosteroids if needed. However, there is less certainty about the use of newer medications such as leukotriene inhibitors, which should be avoided.

Asthma in the elderly

Asthma is common in the elderly, and is often associated with allergy. More severe asthma may be present, with a greater proneness to exacerbations, possibly because of underdiagnosis, undertreatment or poor perception of symptoms. It may be less easy to diagnose asthma in the elderly because these patients may have other diseases that mask the features of asthma, and there may be concomitant chronic obstructive pulmonary disease, particularly in a smoker. Asthma may be associated with the use of medications such as nonsteroidal anti-inflammatory drugs or β-adrenergic blockers. Spirometry may be more difficult to perform in the elderly, but may yield important diagnostic information. In the elderly asthmatic particularly, drugs that may induce or aggravate asthma should be withdrawn. Particular care should be taken in selecting the use of inhaler devices and in giving instructions. If oral corticosteroids are needed, preventive measures against osteoporosis should be considered, including calcium supplements and the use of oestrogen replacement therapy in women and bisphosphonates in men.

Acute severe asthma

PATHOLOGY AND CAUSES

Asthma exacerbations are the major cause of morbidity and mortality in asthma. The pathology of the airways during asthma exacerbations has been extensively described in those patients that have died during a severe asthma exacerbation. The lungs of such patients are grossly hyperinfected, mainly due to the presence of plugs obstructing the small and medium airways. These plugs are composed of inflammatory cells (eosinophils and neutrophils), together with mucus, exuded plasma and proteinaceous material. These plugs have been described sometimes as Curschmann's spiral (condensed mucus of spiral shapes), Creola bodies (airway epithelial cell clusters) or Charcot–Leyden crystals (eosinophils with granule membrane phospholipase). There is usually widespread desquamation of the superficial airway epithelium and the airway wall is grossly thickened with vasodilated bronchial vessels, oedema and a gross infiltration of inflammatory cells, consisting of eosinophils, neutrophils and lymphocytes; in addition, the airway smooth muscle is hypertrophied and in a contracted state. These florid pathological changes can explain the cause of death as acute asphyxia in patients who have died with acute severe asthma. The extent of pathological changes in patients with less severe asthma is not well known but may represent lesser degrees of severity. Examination of sputum specimens from patients with slowly deteriorating asthma, such as that provoked by a controlled reduction of inhaled corticosteroid therapy, shows an increase in eosinophilic and neutrophilic inflammation.

The causes of exacerbations of asthma cannot be determined with any degree of certainty in many cases, but in a large number, there is clinical evidence of an upper respiratory tract infection, usually viral, prior to the exacerbation. In schoolchildren, a respiratory virus can be isolated from nasal washings in as many as 80 per cent of all exacerbations, and 50 per cent of all viruses detected were rhinoviruses. There is little doubt that these viruses can induce an inflammatory response in the airways of patients with asthma. For example, a rhinovirus inoculation into the nose of asthmatic patients causes the levels of eosinophils cationic protein, a marker of eosinophils having been activated, and of interleukin-8 to be increased in nasal lavages. In addition, inflammatory changes in the lower airways are also observed, with accumulation of lymphocytes and eosinophils in the airway submucosa. Such an effect may occur through the release of chemokines (such as eotaxin and RANTES). Experimental work also indicates that rhinovirus infection in an allergic asthmatic potentiates the effect of an allergen exposure, with an increased late asthmatic response and bronchial hyperresponsiveness.

Exposure to allergens is another factor that causes asthma exacerbations in allergic asthmatics. Often, the case is obvious when the offending allergen is known and exposure recognized by the patient. Offending allergens, such as pollens, have been linked to clusters of asthma exacerbations occurring at the time of thunderstorms in the UK or with the unloading of soybeans in Barcelona port. Much less common causes of exacerbations are related to drugs, such as the inadvertent use of β-adrenergic blocking drugs, or aspirin or non-steroid anti-inflammatory drugs in patients with aspirin-sensitive asthma. There is a potential role for stressful events in inducing asthma exacerbations.

CLINICAL PRESENTATION

Asthmatic patients often have isolated symptoms of asthma that are transient, and subside quickly, or are easily relieved by a couple of puffs of inhaled β-agonist. However, recurrent episodes of asthma symptoms may occur with worsening severity, and the patient may feel incompletely relieved by inhaled β-agonists. These are often a prelude to an acute episode of severe asthma. Acute severe asthma is a potentially life-threatening condition that may progress over a period of days, hours or even minutes.

Clinically, it is characterized by shortness of breath of varying degrees of severity, chest tightness, coughing and inability to speak full sentences. Some patients may not be aware of the degree of severity of an attack of asthma, and may only request medical help at late severe stages. Reliance on peak flow measurements as a measure of asthma severity is better for these patients. In a close examination of severe exacerbations, these were found to be characterized by a gradual fall in peak flow expiratory rates over 5–7 days, followed by a more rapid changes over 2–3 days, with an increase in symptoms and in increased use of rescue β-agonists occurring concomitantly. Sometimes symptoms may precede a fall in peak expiratory flow rate. A severe exacerbation is usually considered as being one associated with a greater than 30 per cent fall in peak expiratory flow rate, although this is a very arbitrary definition.

Management of acute severe asthma starts with the recognition of a worsening of asthma and assessing the severity of the airflow obstruction. It is important to be able to predict when an episode of acute severe asthma may occur, so that early preventive steps can be taken. It has to be recognized that many episodes occur too rapidly for preventive steps to be taken. After the patient has been stabilized, it is important to determine whether the causes or triggers of the attack can be avoided or prevented, and to examine whether future attack can be detected and therefore treated earlier.

Varying degrees of severity of acute asthma may present as follows:

1. Mild to moderate: wheezing or coughing without severe distress, able to hold conversation normally, some degree of shortness of breath, peak flow likely to be within 50 per cent of best value.
2. Moderate to severe: wheezing or coughing with some distress, talking in short sentences or phrases, breathing rate increased and tachycardia, peak flow usually less than 50 per cent predicted, some degree of oxygen desaturation (90–95 per cent).
3. Severe, life-threatening: severe respiratory distress, difficulty in talking, cyanosis of tongue, tired and confused, poor respiratory effort with few

wheezes ('silent chest') and weak breath sounds, tachypnoea, bradycardia and hypotension, peak flow less than 30 per cent predicted, oxygen saturation of less than 90 per cent.

TREATMENT

Treatment of acute severe asthma consists of high-flow oxygen, high doses of inhaled β-agonists and systemic corticosteroids, and hospital admission. Addition of ipratropium bromide to β-agonists provides additional bronchodilator response. Intravenous bronchodilators should be considered in life-threatening situations. Sedatives should be avoided at all costs during treatment of acute severe asthma, except if the patient is ventilated.

For the mild to moderate non-life-threatening episode, this can usually be treated at home. The regular use of a β$_2$-agonist aerosol via a pMDI or DPI, up to four puffs every 2–4 hours may reverse the bronchoconstriction. If a nebulizer is available, this should be used for delivering the β-agonist. Oral prednisolone should be initiated at a dose of 30–40 mg/day for at least 5–7 days, when airways obstruction should disappear. Only if the worsening of the asthma, on the basis of changes in PEFR, is mild, may a doubling of inhaled corticosteroids be tried. In case the attack does not respond to the treatment and there is further deterioration, the patient should consider going straight to hospital for further treatment. Often, such patients are inappropriately prescribed a course of antibiotics rather than intensified asthma treatments. Antibiotics are not indicated in most cases of acute severe asthma.

Treatment of the potentially life-threatening attack in the hospital accident and emergency department includes the administration of oxygen by face mask, nebulized β-agonist with an anticholinergic, repeated 1–2-hourly if needed, oral prednisolone (30–40 mg/day) or intravenous hydrocortisone (100–200 mg/6–8-hourly), the latter if the patient is in respiratory failure or experiences gastrointestinal upsets. A chest radiograph is necessary to exclude a pneumothorax or consolidation. Heart rate, respiratory rate and oxygen saturation should be monitored.

In case of deterioration or non-responsiveness to initial treatments, further nebulized β-agonist may be given, with consideration of administration of intravenous β-agonist or aminophylline. Measurements of arterial blood gas with blood electrolytes and sugar should be considered. The patient must be considered for treatment in the intensive care unit with elective intubation and assisted ventilation if he or she becomes tired with weak respiratory effort or becomes comatose and shows severe hypoxaemia, despite administration of oxygen, with hypercapnia (Po$_2$ <8 kPa, Pco$_2$ >6 kPa).

The accompanying figures from the British Thoracic Society's guidelines are summaries of the management of acute severe asthma in adults (Figure 6.3), and the treatment of those aged 5–15 years (Figure 6.4). The principles of management are similar in each situation.

Recognition and assessment in hospital

Features of acute asthma

- Peak expiratory flow (PEF) ≤50 per cent of predicted or best
- Cannot complete sentences in one breath
- Respirations ≥25 breaths/min
- Pulse >110 beats/min

Life-threatening features

- PEF <33 per cent of predicted or best
- Silent chest, cyanosis, or feeble respiratory effort
- Bradycardia or hypotension
- Exhaustion, confusion, or coma

If Sao_2 <92 per cent or a patient has **any life-threatening** features, measure arterial blood gases.

Blood gas markers of a very severe, life-threatening attack:

- Normal (5–6 kPa, 36–45 mmHg) or high $Paco_2$
- Severe hypoxia: Pao_2 <8 kPa (60 mmHg) irrespective of treatment with oxygen
- A low pH (or high H^+)

No other investigations are needed for immediate management.

Caution
Patients with severe or life-threatening attacks may not be distressed and may not have all these abnormalities. The presence of any should alert the doctor

1 Immediate treatment

- Oxygen 40–60 per cent (CO_2 retention is not usually aggravated by oxygen therapy in asthma)
- Salbutamol 5 mg or terbutaline 10 mg via an oxygen-driven nebulizer
- Prednisolone tables 30–60 mg or intravenous hydrocortisone 200 mg or both if very ill
- No sedative of any kind
- Chest radiograph to exclude pneumothorax

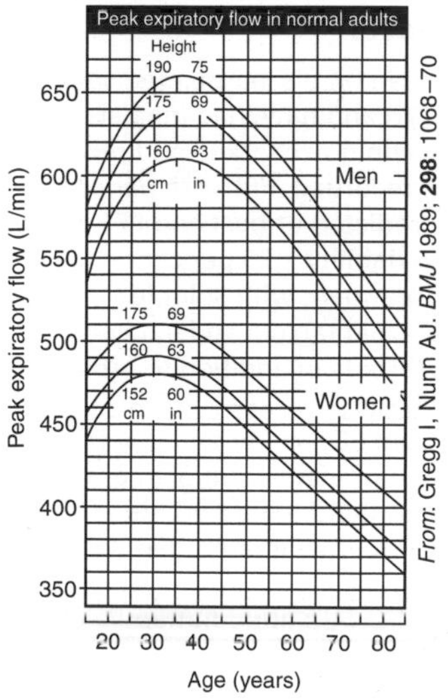

IF LIFE-THREATENING FEATURES ARE PRESENT:

- Add ipratropium 0.5 mg to the nebulized β-agonist
- Give intravenous aminophylline 250 mg over 20 min or salbutamol or terbutaline 250 µg over 10 min. Do not give bolus aminophylline to patients already taking oral theophyllines

2 Subsequent management

IF PATIENT IS IMPROVING CONTINUE:

- 40–60 per cent oxygen
- Prednisolone 30–60 mg daily or intravenous hydrocortisone 200 mg 6-hourly
- Nebulized β-agonist 4-hourly

IF PATIENT IS NOT IMPROVING AFTER 15–30 MINUTES:

- Continue oxygen and steroids
- Give nebulized β-agonist more frequently, up to every 15–30 min
- Add ipratropium 0.5 mg to nebulizer and repeat 6 hourly until patient is improving

IF PATIENT IS STILL NOT IMPROVING GIVE:

- Aminophylline infusion (small patient 750 mg/24 hours, large patient 1500 mg/24 hours); monitor blood concentrations if it is continued for over 24 hours
- Salbutamol or terbutaline infusion as an alternative to aminophylline

3 Monitoring treatment

- Repeat measurement of PEF 15–30 min after starting treatment
- Oximetry: maintain Sao_2 >92 per cent
- Repeat blood gas measurements within 2 hours of starting treatment if

  – initial Pao_2 <8 kPa (60 mmHg) unless subsequent Sao_2 >92 per cent
  – $Paco_2$ normal or raised
  – patient deteriorates
- Chart PEF before and after giving nebulized or inhaled β-agonists and at least 4 times daily throughout hospital stay

Transfer patient to the intensive care unit accompanied by a doctor prepared to intubate if there is:

- Deteriorating PEF, worsening or persisting hypoxia, or hypercapnia
- Exhaustion, feeble respirations, confusion or drowsiness
- Coma or respiratory arrest

4 When discharged from hospital, patients should have:

- Been on discharge medication for 24 hour and *have had inhaler technique checked and recorded*
- PEF >75 per cent of predicted or best and PEF diurnal variability <25 per cent *unless discharge is agreed with respiratory physician*
- Treatment with *oral and inhaled steroids* in addition to bronchodilators
- Own PEF meter and *written self-management plan*
- GP follow-up arranged *within 1 week*
- Follow-up appointment in respiratory clinic *within 4 weeks*

Also

- Determine reason(s) for exacerbation and admission
- Send details of admission, discharge and potential best PEF to GP.

From: Gregg I, Nunn AJ. BMJ 1989; 298: 1068–70

Peak expiratory flow in normal adults

Figure 6.3
Management of acute severe asthma in adults. (Reproduced with permission of the BMJ Publishing Group from the British Thoracic Society (1997) *Thorax* 52 **(suppl. 1)**.)

Recognition of acute severe asthma

- Too breathless to talk
- Too breathless to feed
- Respirations ≥40 breaths/min
- Pulse >120 beats/min
- PEF ≤50 per cent predicted or best

Life-threatening features
- PEF <33 per cent predicted or best
- Cyanosis, silent chest, or poor respiratory effort
- Fatigue or exhaustion
- Agitation or reduced level of consciousness

No other investigations are needed for immediate management

Blood gas estimations are rarely helpful in deciding initial management in children

Caution:
Children with severe attacks may not appear distressed; assessment in the very young may be difficult. The presence of any of these features should alert the doctor.

Management of a severe asthma attack

1 Immediate treatment
- High flow oxygen via face mask
- Salbutamol 5 mg or terbutaline 10 mg via an oxygen-driven nebulizer (half doses in very young children)
- Prednisolone 1–2 mg/kg body weight orally (maximum 40 mg)

IF LIFE-THREATENING FEATURES ARE PRESENT:

- Give intravenous aminophylline 5 mg/kg over 20 min followed by maintenance infusion, 1 mg/kg per h; omit the loading dose if child already receiving oral theophyllines
- Give intravenous hydrocortisone 100 mg 6-hourly

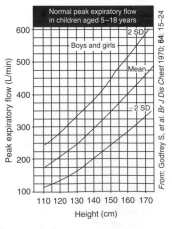

*From: Godfrey S, et al. Br J Dis Chest 1970; **64**: 15–24*

- Add ipratropium 0.25 mg to nebulized β-agonist (0.125 mg in very young children)
- Pulse oximetry is helpful in assessing response to treatment An Sao_2 ≤92 per cent may indicate the need for chest radiography

2 Subsequent management
IF PATIENT IS IMPROVING CONTINUE:
- High-flow oxygen
- Prednisolone 1–2 mg/kg daily (maximum 40 mg/day)
- Nebulized β-agonist 4-hourly

IF PATIENT IS NOT IMPROVING AFTER 15–30 MINUTES:
- Continue oxygen and steroids
- Give nebulized β-agonist more frequently, up to every 30 min
- Add ipratropium to nebulizer and repeat 6-hourly until improvement starts

IF PATIENT IS STILL NOT IMPROVING GIVE:
- Aminophylline infusion (1 mg/kg per h); monitor blood concentrations if continued for over 24 hours

3 Monitoring treatment
- Repeat PEF measurement 15–30 min after starting treatment (if appropriate)
- Oximetry: maintain Sao_2 >92 per cent

- Chart PEF if appropriate before and after the child inhales β-agonists and at least 4 times daily throughout hospital stay

4 Transfer to the intensive care unit accompanied by a doctor prepared to intubate if there is:
- Deteriorating PEF, worsening or persisting hypoxia, or hypercapnia
- Exhaustion, feeble respirations, confusion or drowsiness
- Coma or respiratory arrest

5 When discharged from hospital patients should have:
- Been on discharge medication for 24 h and have had inhaler technique checked and recorded
- If recorded, PEF >75 per cent of predicted or best and PEF diurnal variability <25 per cent
- Treatment with soluble steroid tablets and inhaled steroids in addition to bronchodilators
- Own PEF meter and if appropriate self-management plan or written instructions for parents
- GP follow-up arranged within 1 week
- Follow-up appointment in clinic within 4 weeks

Figure 6.4
Management of acute severe asthma in those aged 5–15 years. (Reproduced with permission of the BMJ Publishing Group from the British Thoracic Society (1997) *Thorax* **52 (suppl. 1).**)

MANAGEMENT AFTER THE ACUTE EPISODE

Following recovery from the acute episode, the patient is considered for discharge from hospital when peak flows have recovered to more than 75 per cent of predicted or of best pre-attack peak flows, and there is no longer evidence of respiratory failure, with oxygen saturation >95 per cent while breathing room air. Medications on discharge should include a continuing but reducing course of oral prednisolone and regular inhaled bronchodilators. Prophylactic medication should be introduced or, if taken by the patient prior to the attack, it should be continued and may be increased. For example, inhaled corticosteroid therapy may be increased in an attempt to prevent further recurrence. This opportunity must be taken to reinforce adherence to anti-inflammatory therapy and to review inhaler technique. Possible non-compliance to treatments must be investigated. A written self-management plan should be instituted for early detection and institution of treatment for possible future attacks, with the use of an asthma diary, preferably with peak flow measurements to document airways lability. In some special circumstances, the episode of asthma may occur very rapidly and can be life-threatening, and may not be prevented by preventive therapies. The use of self-injections of intramuscular adrenaline at the start of these attacks must be considered, and the patient trained in self-injections; in this case also, it is important to review the quickest access to emergency treatment for this particular patient.

Although triggers such as upper respiratory tract virus infections (rhinoviruses, coronaroviruses) and allergens may be indentified as causing the acute episode of asthma in some patients, there are currently no ways of preventing the effects of these triggers. Administration of anti-flu vaccine in the autumn is recommended for all asthmatic patients. Usually, a doubling of anti-inflammatory therapy (for example, inhaled corticosteroid therapy) at the earliest sign of an attack is proposed for patients in a self-management plan, despite the lack of evidence as to the efficacy of this treatment.

Following an acute attack of asthma treated in hospital, patients should be reviewed regularly. In addition, patients recovering from an acute attack of asthma at home should also be considered for referral to a local asthma specialist centre for review.

Asthma in infants and children

7

Andrew Bush

'Asthma' in the infant and younger child

When it comes to asthma, the infant and the younger child cannot be regarded as adults in miniature. The problems are so different that 'asthma syndrome' may be a better term. This chapter begins with a discussion of the differential diagnosis, which is more extensive than in adult asthma. Subsequently the different pathophysiology and treatment approaches will be discussed. At the end of the chapter, the controversy about the use of the word 'asthma' will be revisited.

DIFFERENTIAL DIAGNOSIS

It is important to be sure that you know what the parents mean by wheeze; some will mean a high-pitched expiratory whistle, some will mean a bubbling, crackling upper airway noise, some will mean a nasal stuffiness and some will mean stridor. The younger the wheezing child, the more important it is that other diagnoses be considered, but it is also true at all ages that 'asthma' may not respond to treatment because the diagnosis is wrong. There are specific points in the history (Box 7.1) and physical examination (Box 7.2) which should suggest an alternative diagnosis. In most cases, after a careful history and physical examination, possibly supplemented by a chest radiograph, a trial of treatment will be given. Physiological measurements, the bedrock of management in the older child, are usually not available in routine clinical practice in babies and toddlers.

Easily the most common cause of cough and wheeze which is misdiagnosed as asthma in infants is prolonged post-infective (usually post-viral) cough. The cardinal rule to prevent mislabelling a child as asthmatic is to keep trying to reduce treatment once symptoms have disappeared. If this rule is not followed, transient symptoms will be overtreated, and inhaled steroids continued in the erroneous belief that it is treatment, not the passage of time, which has caused symptoms to disappear.

Box 7.1
Specific pointers to be sought in the clinical history which might suggest a diagnosis other than asthma

- Are the child/family really describing wheeze?
- Symptoms disappearing during sleep.
- Upper airway symptoms – snoring, rhinitis, sinusitis.
- Symptoms from the first day of life.
- Very sudden onset of symptoms.
- Chronic moist cough/sputum production.
- Worse wheeze or irritable after feed, worse when lying down, vomiting, choking on feeds.
- Any feature of a systemic immunodeficiency.
- Continuous, unremitting or worsening symptoms.

Box 7.2
Specific physical signs to be sought which should prompt consideration of an alternative diagnosis

- Digital clubbing, signs of weight loss, failure to thrive.
- Upper airway disease – enlarged tonsils and adenoids, prominent rhinitis, nasal polyps.
- Unusually severe chest deformity (Harrison's sulcus, barrel chest).
- Fixed monophonic wheeze.
- Stridor (monophasic or biphasic).
- Asymmetric wheeze.
- Signs of cardiac or systemic disease.

The differential diagnosis of childhood wheeze is given in Box 7.3. The classical presentation of cystic fibrosis with recurrent chest infections, foul diarrhoea, a voracious appetite and failure to thrive in infancy is well known. However, there are numerous traps into which general practitioners and hospital doctors fall with monotonous regularity. Diagnosis is frequently delayed (up to 15 per cent into adult life); 10–15 per cent of children are pancreatic sufficient, and will thrive; at least at first, respiratory problems may be mild. Depressingly, digital clubbing is often not sought in children; gross clubbing is not infrequent at late presentation, implying that it has been missed repeatedly. The golden rule should be to perform a sweat test in any child in whom either the doctor or the family consider cystic fibrosis to be a possibility, no matter how remote.

Endobronchial foreign body is easily treatable if diagnosed, and disastrous if missed. It should be considered even if the infant is too young to put objects in the mouth; an older sibling may helpfully do it for them. Obvious clues are

- Upper airway disease – adenotonsillar hypertrophy, rhinosinusitis, postnasal drip.
- Congenital structural bronchial disease – complete cartilage rings, cysts, webs.
- Bronchial/tracheal compression – vascular rings and sling, enlarged cardiac chamber, lymph nodes enlarged by tuberculosis or lymphoma.
- Endobronchial disease – foreign body, tumour.
- Oesophageal/swallowing problems – reflux, incoordinate swallow, laryngeal cleft or tracheo-oesophageal fistula.
- Causes of pulmonary suppuration – cystic fibrosis, primary ciliary dyskinesia, any systemic immunodeficiency, including agammaglobulinaemia, severe combined immuno-deficiency.
- Psychological – vocal cord dysfunction, habit/honk cough.
- Miscellaneous – bronchopulmonary dysplasia, congenital or acquired tracheomalacia, pulmonary oedema.

Box 7.3
Differential diagnosis of asthma in children

the onset of symptoms in a previously well child after a choking fit; but suspicion also should be aroused if the history is of very sudden onset. Parents should always be asked specifically about the possibility of foreign body, because the history may not be volunteered. There may be obvious asymmetrical wheeze, or no physical signs. If foreign body is suspected, urgent referral for consideration of bronchoscopy is mandatory. The penalty for missing the diagnosis may be severe pneumonia, lung abscess or bronchiectasis.

Oesophageal disease may present as wheeze. The most common consideration is gastro-oesophageal reflux, which may cause or coexist with wheeze. Easy vomiting and repeated posseting are obvious pointers; but this diagnosis should also be considered if the wheeze is present every day, worse after meals, and the child is irritable and difficult to feed. Dyscoordinate swallowing due to neuromuscular problems (often cerebral palsy) and H-type tracheo-oesophageal fistula and laryngeal cleft are less usual considerations.

Congenital causes of wheeze should be considered, in particular if the symptoms started on the first day of life, which asthma never does. These include bronchogenic cyst, the numerous types of vascular ring, complete cartilage rings, subglottic stenosis and tracheo-bronchomalacia. Another problem which may present in the first year of life is primary ciliary dyskinesia, previously known as Kartagener's syndrome. Classically, the child has rhinitis present every day, but only 50 per cent of patients have dextrocardia.

Box 7.4
Diagnostic tests that may need to be considered in refractory asthma/infant wheeze

- Suspected oesophageal disease – pH probe, barium swallow, tube oesophagram, oesophagoscopy.
- Suspected upper airway disease – polysomnography, RAST tests (radiograph of postnasal space is rarely useful).
- Suspected cystic fibrosis – sweat test, nasal potentials, genotype, stool elastase, faecal fat.
- Suspected primary ciliary dyskinesia – saccharine test, nasal ciliary motility, electron microscopy including orientation studies, nasal and exhaled nitric oxide.
- Suspected systemic immunodeficiency – immunoglobulins and subclasses, vaccine antibodies, lymphocyte subsets, lymphocyte and neutrophil function tests, HIV test.
- Suspected structural airway disease – fibreoptic bronchoscopy.
- Suspected tuberculosis – Heaf test, fibreoptic bronchoscopy and/or gastric lavage, combined with culture and polymerase chain reaction (PCR).
- Suspected cardiovascular disease – echocardiogram, barium swallow to exclude a vascular ring or pulmonary artery sling, angiography.
- Suspected bronchiectasis – high-resolution CT scan, investigations for local or systemic immunodeficiency.

Recurrent pulmonary oedema may present as wheeze; causes include patent arterial duct, ventricular septal defect and cardiomyopathy. Finally, chronic sputum production, or more usually a chronic moist cough, should also result in a more detailed diagnostic evaluation. Although the most common cause is a postnasal drip, and asthma can certainly be associated with sputum production, the more prominent the cough, and the less wheeze is a feature, the more the physician should be careful not to miss another diagnosis. Bronchiectasis due to cystic fibrosis or other immunodeficiency is not rare in childhood, and if the diagnosis is missed, catastrophic and irreversible deterioration in lung function may result. An outline of useful investigations is given in Box 7.4.

WHAT DOES WHEEZING IN INFANCY MEAN?

Infant wheeze is not miniature adult asthma; in most cases, there is no evidence of inflammation, and bronchial hyperreactivity is not a prerequisite for wheeze. The whole mindset has to be different, or important treatment errors will be made.

Importance of airway development

A number of different studies have emphasized the importance of prenatal events, such as exposure to parental smoking, or the parents' atopic status or the presence of maternal hypertension during the pregnancy, in subsequent wheezing. These studies strongly suggest an important effect of the intrauterine environment on airway growth. Three prospective studies in Perth (Australia), Tucson (USA) and Boston (USA) have emphasized the importance of anatomical (developmental) factors in infant wheezing in cohorts of babies recruited either before or soon after birth. Lung function was measured using a variety of techniques before the infants had ever had any respiratory symptoms. During follow-up, some of these babies developed wheezing lower respiratory tract illnesses. This group of babies had evidence of airflow obstruction and impaired lung function before their first wheezing illness. In other words, these babies wheezed because of a long pre-existing abnormality of the airway, and not because they had been 'normal' but had become infected with a particularly virulent virus. The most likely explanation is that infants who wheeze, in particular with viral colds, do so because their lower airway diameters are less than normal because of impaired airway development in the second half of pregnancy. Any viral infection leading to mucosal oedema or inflammation would be more likely to narrow the lumen enough to cause wheezing. This explanation would predict that, as these babies grow older, that they would wheeze less as the airway diameter increases with growth, and this is exactly what happens (see p. 120). Further evidence that events occurring prior to birth determine the outcome from respiratory diseases comes from other observations. First, studies from England and Australia have shown that there is no relationship between bronchial hyperreactivity and early viral-induced wheezing. Second, children with atopic asthma (wheezing with viral colds and between colds with typical stimuli such as cold air, exercise and furry pets) had increased numbers of eosinophils in bronchoalveolar lavage fluid, whereas those who wheezed only with viral colds did not; and, finally, a randomized, double-blind, placebo-controlled trial of inhaled steroids in infants with virus-associated wheeze showed no benefit. Thus, viral-associated wheeze is a different entity from atopic asthma, and thus, by inference, needs a different treatment approach.

The effect of atopy

Another important influence that interacts with intrauterine growth is atopy. This interaction may be important at different levels. First, maternal (more than paternal) atopic status is predictive of atopy in the child. Second, there is some evidence that the fetus may develop atopic sensitization during the second half of the pregnancy, not merely to maternal food allergens, but also to aeroallergens. Third, ingested maternal food allergens (in particular cow's milk) may cross into the breast milk of the lactating woman. Fourth, there appears to be a window of particular vulnerability to allergic sensitization in the first few months of life; for example, sensitivity to birch pollen in Scandinavia is much higher if the first 6 months of life overlap with the birch pollen season.

There is a curious interaction between family order and atopy. Thus, the more older siblings in the family, the less likely the baby is to become atopic. One suggestion is that early and repeated viral infections unwittingly transmitted to the baby by the older children may have the beneficial effect of switching the Th0 uncommitted T-lymphocyte to a Th1 antiviral pattern, rather than the Th2 atopic/allergic cytokine profile. In favour of this was the finding of a fall in total IgE after viral infections which did not cause wheeze in the Tucson study. Furthermore, evidence of previous gastrointestinal infection or measles is more common in those who do not have asthma, implying a beneficial effect of early infections. For the moment, the validity of the observation is unchallenged, but the explanation remains unclear.

Whereas wheezing with viral colds is no more prevalent in atopic babies, wheeze between colds is related to atopy. There is some evidence that interval symptoms are more predictive of the persistence of symptoms into the pattern of true asthma, and may be more responsive to inhaled corticosteroids. One problem with many studies on the response to therapy in this age group has been that all wheeze has been lumped together, be it wheeze purely with viral colds and no interval symptoms, or daily wheeze irrespective of infection. It seems likely, but unproven, that the pathophysiology may be quite different, with the atopic wheezers more likely to have eosinophil mediated, T-cell-driven airway inflammation, and those wheezing just with colds having reduced airway calibre on a developmental basis.

Prognosis for infant wheeze

A prospective follow-up study in Leicester showed that half of all atopic infants, and two-thirds of those who were non-atopic, who wheezed in the first 2 years of life, were asymptomatic at school age. Other prospective studies have confirmed that most wheezing infants will improve as they get older. Furthermore, an Australian study which followed children from age 7 to age 35 years showed clearly that those who were still wheezing with viral colds, even at age 7, had completely normal lung function in adult life, irrespective of whether they had been treated with inhaled corticosteroids or not. Those with symptoms between colds did, however, have persistent airflow obstruction, the severity of which was proportional to the severity of their childhood disease. These follow-up data also need to be considered when planning treatment guidelines for wheezing infants. First, many wheezy infants do not have airway inflammation and do not need inhaled steroids; second, many will get better whatever is done, and stepping down treatment is essential when control of symptoms has been achieved.

THE PHARMACOLOGICAL APPROACH

The current model for the older child

There is evidence that T-lymphocyte-driven, eosinophil-mediated airway inflammation, if left untreated, will lead to airway remodelling and fixed airflow obstruction. In adult asthmatics, early treatment with inhaled cortico-steroids leads to a better treatment response; however, the evidence in a paediatric population is less rigorous. A non-randomized Danish study in children of mean age 6 years demonstrated that there was a dose–response effect, such that the longer the duration of asthma symptoms beyond 2 years prior to starting inhaled steroids, the worse the long-term lung function. A Dutch study, again comparing inhaled corticosteroids plus β_2-agonist versus placebo plus β_2-agonist, showed that airway reactivity declined only in the inhaled corticosteroid group. Of concern was that it never normalized, did not reach a plateau even after 2 years of treatment and worsened again when the inhaled steroids were stopped. Thus inhaled steroids did not, in this group, appear to be disease-modifying. Furthermore, some of the β_2-agonist group did as well as the inhaled steroid group. There has not been a corres-ponding study in small infants, although it is that of concern that features of airway remodelling have been seen even in young children. Whether this remodelling is either truly irreversible or clinically significant is not clear. In summary, the evidence for early and aggressive use of inhaled steroids in wheezing infants is not nearly as strong as it is in older children and adults.

Step one: intermittent treatment

Many young infants with symptoms triggered solely by viral colds do not respond particularly well to any treatment. My practice in infants under 18 months is to try both ipratropium bromide and β_2-agonist, to see which (if either) works. In most cases, a mask and spacer will be used, in which case up to 10 puffs up to 4-hourly should be administered. In the unlikely event that nebulized ipratropium is used, the first dose should be administered under supervision to check that paradoxical bronchoconstriction is not a problem. The older the child, the less inclined am I to use ipratropium.

Oral β_2-agonist is generally not efficacious. However, there are a few infants with mild wheeze whose families say they respond well to this medi-cation, and even fewer physicians who can honestly say that they have never prescribed oral β_2-agonist.

Prophylactic medication (Steps 2–4) is usually prescribed if:

1. there are interval symptoms necessitating rescue medication more than an arbitrary number of times per week (usually 3–4);
2. interval symptoms are interfering with lifestyle; and
3. (more controversially) there are severe symptoms with viral colds. The evi-dence for and against this indication will be reviewed below.

Step two: non-steroidal anti-inflammatory agents

Two main classes of drugs have been used; these are the oral antihistamines and inhaled cromolyns, most usually disodium cromoglycate (DSCG). The use of all these agents is controversial, and many bypass this step altogether. Oral ketotifen has been used with variable benefit in wheezing infants, but is being used less and less. The place of DSCG in wheezing infants was the subject of a recent large, double-blind Dutch study. This showed clearly that DSCG was no better than placebo for the groups. A few individuals may do well with DSCG, probably particularly if they are highly atopic, and the medication is so safe that there is little to be lost from a short therapeutic trial, typically 2 months. Although one group showed some benefit in infants wheezing secondary to premature birth, most have found DSCG of limited benefit in this infancy. It has the further disadvantage of needing to be given 3–4 times per day. In most instances, step 2 will be bypassed in infants.

Step three: the use of inhaled corticosteroids

The most popular anti-inflammatory agents used in infants are inhaled corticosteroids. As discussed above, the pathophysiology of wheeze in infants may be very different, with developmental factors predominating over airway inflammation. Thus there is no reason to prescribe inhaled corticosteroids for all wheezing infants. However, a therapeutic trial of inhaled steroids for a strictly limited time period is quite legitimate. Three inhaled steroids are currently available: beclomethasone dipropionate (BDP), budesonide (BUD) and fluticasone propionate (FP). FP has not been licensed for use with those under age 5 years, and the balance of the evidence is that BUD has a lower risk of systemic side-effects. I give a trial of relatively high dose BUD (400 μg twice daily) for 2 months, to try to determine whether the wheezing process is steroid sensitive. If there is complete resolution of symptoms, then I stop the steroid altogether. If symptoms recur, and respond again to inhaled steroids, I consider that a diagnosis of asthma has been established, and I reduce the dose briskly to determine the minimum dose needed to control symptoms. If there is absolutely no change in symptoms after the therapeutic trial, I would discontinue inhaled steroids, and consider other approaches (see p. 122) and review the diagnosis. The step-down approach as soon as control has been obtained remains very important. Finally, there is little evidence that commencing high-dose inhaled steroids at the onset of symptoms of a viral cold is of any benefit, nor that the practice of recommending the family to double the dose of inhaled steroids with viral colds is helpful either.

A further reason for caution is the possibility of side-effects. Inhaled steroids in general have an impressive safety profile. There are always concerns about linear growth, adrenal function, bone density and cataract formation in the older child. These are discussed on pp. 71–3. The particular issue in the infant is the theoretical possibility of interference with lung growth. The first 3 years of life are the time of alveolar multiplication. In neonatal animals, systemic steroids inhibit alveolar multiplication. It may be wrong to extrapolate from systemic steroids in the rat to inhaled steroids in the infant; however, possible alveolar underdevelopment cannot be excluded in humans. This as another reason why inhaled steroids should be used appropriately.

Step four: when inhaled corticosteroids fail

At this point, a number of steps need to be carried out. The child will usually have been referred to a paediatrician with a special interest in respiratory medicine. A review of other diagnostic possibilities needs to be performed. A basic minimum of investigations should be carried out, even if there seems little doubt about the diagnosis. This would include a sweat test, immunoglobulins and immunoglobulin subclasses, the response to vaccine antibodies, skin-prick or RAST tests to common allergens (house dust mite, cat, dog, grass pollen) and a pH study. The respiratory nurse should re-check the techniques being used with the drug-delivery device. The question of adherence to treatment should be explored sensitively with the parents, and the general practitioner contacted to see how many prescriptions have actually been dispensed. A review of environmental factors which could be exacerbating symptoms should be performed. Another possibility is parental misperception of the severity of the symptoms. In general, the doctor who thinks he knows more than the mother is riding for a fall; just occasionally, due to extreme overanxiety, or even as a variant of the Münchausen by proxy syndrome, the mother exaggerates the child's symptoms. Clues may come if there is a marked disparity between the perception of mother and doctor (and especially mother and nurse) if the child is brought up to hospital as an emergency. The help of an experienced community nurse to assess the child in the home may resolve these doubts. Occasionally an admission to hospital and assessment by experienced paediatric nurses may be needed. If, after this process, it is clear that the only room for manoeuvre is pharmacotherapy, then a number of options are available. A trial of salmeterol (not licensed for use in this age group) may be worthwhile, and there is some evidence that increasing the dose as high as $100\,\mu g$ twice daily is useful. If theophylline is used, then the physician needs to be alert to possible drug interactions, particularly with erythromycin. Although there have been concerns about possible behavioural and cognitive disturbances in children on theophylline, these are probably rare, albeit distressing when they do occur.

If these relatively straightforward options fail, then other, more invasive possibilities include: alternate-day or even daily oral steroids; the use of subcutaneous terbutaline; intravenous immunoglobulin; or even a steroid-sparing agent such as methotrexate or cyclosporin. There is not much experience with these options in infants.

The fat, happy wheezer

This is a common phrase to describe the infant who is in no distress and plays happily while making loud wheezing noises. Although the child may be happy, the family, exhausted by seemingly endless sleepless nights, is often most unhappy. Sometimes the noises largely disappear when the child is asleep, implying that perhaps tracheo-bronchomalacia is the underlying pathophysiology. Trials of simple treatment (inhaled anticholinergics and β-agonists) usually fail, and a search for an underlying treatable condition is unsuccessful. This is often an insoluble paediatric conundrum; reassurance, particularly about the long-term prognosis, may be all that can be offered. It is important to ensure that any treatment is not worse than the problem.

How should medications be administered?

The oral route is not recommended, despite its convenience. The choice lies between a spacer and a nebulizer. Children over 3 years of age can usually use a mouthpiece, but younger infants will need a soft face mask. The ideal drug-delivery device would be cheap, convenient, quick to use, easy to carry around and requiring no maintenance. The nebulizer is thus outperformed on every count; if a nebulizer is to be used ahead of a mask and spacer, this requires careful justification.

A variety of spacers have been used in children, but there is a paucity of good drug deposition data. The still more serious lack in the literature is information about what devices are actually most useful at home, rather than in the asthma laboratory. It is important to allow parental choice. The small aerochamber is less efficient than the larger-volume spacers, but its portability makes it popular with families. The spacer should be washed weekly in ordinary household detergent, not rinsed, and left to drip dry. This reduces electrostatic deposition of medication. When the aerosol is used, there should be no delay between activating the aerosol and the child inhaling from the device; if the inhaler is activated and the infant then has to be pursued around the room, the medication will have been lost by the time he or she has been caught. If multiple activations are required, then the inhaler must be shaken and the child must inhale from the spacer between each activation.

If the family wants to use a nebulizer, it is vital to emphasize that there is no evidence that drug delivery is superior. Although rare infants will do better with nebulized budesonide rather than an inhaled steroid, most will be equally well managed with a spacer. If use of a nebulizer is inevitable, then it is important that the child actually has the mask firmly over the mouth and nose; hopefully waving the nebulizer somewhere near the child's face in the hope that he or she will inhale some medication is not useful.

There is no doubt that the inhaled route may be difficult for parents and child. A skilled nurse helps, and it is important to emphasize that a gentle but firm approach will pay off. The child has to realize who is in charge and that the medication will be administered with or without a fight; when this agenda has been set, then the problems usually resolve. It is worth noting, however, that if the child is actually screaming when the spacer is used, drug deposition is reduced not increased, despite the infant's apparent increased ventilation during yelling. Judicious bribery is always helpful. As the child reaches the third birthday, if medication is still needed, he or she should be switched from a mask to a mouthpiece with appropriate training. Finally, the issues for choice of inhaler device in the older child are discussed below.

WHAT ENVIRONMENTAL MANIPULATIONS ARE POSSIBLE?

There is more to asthma treatment than the prescription pad. If low-dose (up to 800 μg/day) inhaled corticosteroid is not working, then detailed consideration of the child's environment is mandatory; and in all asthmatics, some thought beyond pharmacotherapy is always a good idea. Cigarette smoking by adults in front of children is child abuse. The adverse effects occur during pregnancy, and postnatally. Besides the direct irritant effects of smoking on the airway, the risks of allergic sensitization are increased. No parent ever admits to smoking in front of their child; however, by some mysterious process, their children are actually exposed, as shown by high levels of the stable nicotine metabolite, cotinine, in the child's urine. That parents should not smoke is indubitable; how to persuade them, and help them to stop, is quite another matter.

Allergen avoidance should preferably be preceded by a precise allergy diagnosis. This is difficult in the young infant, in whom skin tests may be less reliable than in the older child. Thus often an empirical approach is taken. Allergen avoidance is unlikely to help symptoms associated with viral cold. However, symptoms between colds, particularly in the atopic infant and particularly if they are difficult to control with pharmacotherapy, may mean that a look at possible adverse environmental influences may be worthwhile, if the family is sufficiently motivated.

House dust mite avoidance is relatively straightforward. The mattress, duvet and (when used) the pillow should be covered in mite-impermeable cases. Bed linen should be washed at 60°C. The carpet should be taken out of the bedroom. Soft toys should be kept in a cupboard; if it is inevitable that the child has a teddy bear in bed, then the bear should be put in the deep freeze for 24 hours once a month to kill mites (be sure the bear is thawed out before it goes back into the bed).

Pets are a major bugbear. In most British households, they are considered to be far more important than children. The major arguments for not getting rid of the cat or dog are on the lines of 'We have always had one, and his asthma only started when he was 6 months old'; and 'We got rid of the cat for 3 weeks and he was no better'. Neither excludes pet sensitivity as a cause of symptoms. In a study of serial subacute inhalant allergen challenges in adults, designed not to produce acute changes in lung function, there was evidence of increasing sputum eosinophilia and worsening bronchial hyperreactivity with serial challenges. Furthermore, the major cat allergen, *Fel d1*, persists in the environment for many months after having got rid of the cat. The burden of allergen can be reduced by washing the cat weekly; I decline to believe that many pet owners will do this long term.

Other factors blamed are food allergy and air pollution. Generally, food exclusion does not work in asthma; the parents will usually have tried and failed before the child is brought to the doctor. Significant food allergy is generally very obvious. The exception is in Asian asthmatics, whose symptoms may be made worse by Coca-Cola, very cold drinks and fried food. There is clear-cut evidence that acute changes in environmental factors can worsen asthma, but no evidence that, for the majority of asthmatics, air pollution is an important factor in their symptoms. Indeed, one study showed equal asthma prevalence in those breathing the pure air of the Scottish isles as in those in inner-city Glasgow. Comparisons between the populations of former East and West Germany showed more evidence of atopic asthma in the wealthier West, despite the heavy industrial pollution of East Germany.

THE DIAGNOSIS OF ASTHMA

Cough-variant asthma is a genuine entity, but doctors, having initially been reluctant ever to give a child with cough but no wheeze a diagnosis of asthma, are now overdiagnosing cough-variant asthma. Cough as a sole symptom in community-based, questionnaire surveys is poorly predictive of asthma. Clearly, the predictive value of cough as a symptom of asthma will vary with the setting in which the question is asked. The more prominent the cough, and the less the wheeze, the more reluctant am I to accept a diagnosis of asthma. A really thorough review of other diagnoses is essential (see p. 127), with particular thought to gastro-oesophageal reflux and postnasal drip. If, after such a review, asthma still seems a likely diagnosis and the child is too young to perform pulmonary function tests, then I will proceed straight to step 3 (above) and give a therapeutic trial of inhaled corticosteroids (BUD, 400 μg twice daily). Alternatively, a trial of bronchodilators can be given, particularly if the symptoms are relatively minor. Oral steroid trials are not recommended in this age group; they are non-specific, treating adenoidal hypertrophy and rhinosinusitis, and also there is a risk of side-effects, albeit small. Since so many causes of childhood cough are transient and reversible (post-viral and post-mycoplasma, for example), if the symptoms disappear it is essential to stop treatment and only give the child a diagnosis of asthma if symptoms recur and respond again to inhaled steroids. In the older child who can do lung function tests, a period of home peak flow monitoring, or a shuttle exercise test, or response of peak flow to bronchodilator should be carried out to determine whether there is truly variable airflow obstruction. If none of these tests is positive, the diagnosis of asthma is unlikely.

There is epidemiological evidence that many children with chronic cough represent a different group from the true asthmatics, with a lower prevalence of atopy and a good prognosis. Some undoubtedly go on to develop true asthma, but this is the exception. Perhaps we should be more ready to accept a diagnosis of chronic non-specific cough and offer reassurance not medication to the group of coughing children who do not respond to asthma treatments.

My infant wheezes – does he have asthma?

This is one of the most vexed of all questions in paediatrics, and the right answer probably depends on who is asking the question and for what purpose. The real trouble with the question is that the definition of asthma has been hijacked; the perfectly acceptable definition 'wheeze and/or cough in a setting where asthma is likely and other, rarer diagnoses have been excluded' has been altered to include underlying pathological concepts of airway inflammation. By the new definition, most infants wheezers do NOT have asthma, because they do not have airway inflammation. Therefore, the term 'asthma syndrome' is preferred, emphasizing the different pathophysiological mechanisms of wheeze. While the purists argue, what the parents want to know is whether their child will grow up continuing to have symptoms of asthma and requiring to take treatment. At the moment, although a number of sophisticated tests have been proposed, none is predictive for the individual. The more severe the symptoms, and the stronger the evidence of atopy, the more likely it is that symptoms will persist into mid-childhood and beyond.

Special issues in the older child with asthma

The current BTS asthma guidelines include children over age five with adults, thus proceeding from a non-evidence-based position to one of total folly. A 6-year-old is not a miniature 20-year-old in any sense worth discussing, and should not be treated as such.

DIAGNOSIS

Most of the diagnostic considerations listed earlier are equally relevant in the older age group. Most important, different from infants, and done much less well than by adults' physicians, is to obtain lung function evidence of variable airflow obstruction (see above) and benefit from treatment. It is still depressingly common to be referred a child with 'non-responsive asthma' who has had no lung function measurements, has been placed on a huge cocktail of medications, and in fact does not have asthma at all.

PHARMACOTHERAPY

The prophylactic medication, DSCG, is used less and less even in this age group (with the possible exception of exercise-induced asthma, see p. 129), because studies have shown that asthma control is less good, and side-effects the same as with very low-dose inhaled steroids. There is no paediatric evidence to favour either starting with high-dose inhaled steroids and tapering down, or low-dose steroids and increasing the dose if necessary. Empirically, I adopt both approaches, depending on the presentation. Children with minor symptoms, but sufficient to use a bronchodilator several times per week, can be treated very successfully with no more than 200 μg/day BUD, whereas others with much worse asthma would be started on a higher dose, say 800 μg/day. The importance of seeing the child at least every 3 months, and actively considering whether the time is right to decrease the dose of medication, cannot be overemphasized. Finally, although the leukotriene antagonists have been licensed as first-line preventive therapy in mild to moderate paediatric asthma, there is no evidence that they are safer or better than low-dose inhaled steroids. If they have a role, it will be as an adjunct to inhaled steroids (see below).

CHOICE OF 'ADD-ON' THERAPY

When a moderate dose of inhaled steroid fails to control symptoms, the choices are either greatly increasing the dose or adding on another agent. There is much debate as to where the top of the steroid dose–response curve lies, and it clearly varies between individuals and over time within individuals. It is not clear at what point increasing the dose of steroids is not worthwhile, and when and what should be added in. On balance, if an increase in inhaled steroids to 800 μg/day fails to control symptoms completely, then an add-on medication should be considered. The choices lie between long-acting β_2-agonists, leukotriene receptor antagonists and low-dose theophyllines. There are no comparisons to guide choice, nor any evidence that two of these agents together is of any value. Most trials of salmeterol in significantly symptomatic patients have shown evidence of benefit. The occurrence of tachyphylaxis to its bronchoprotective effects has led to some calling for its use only intermittently, for example on the days the child does sport at school, but this is currently a minority view. The standard dose is 50 μg twice daily, but there is some evidence that a minority of children may benefit from doubling the dose. There are, unfortunately, no paediatric trials of leukotriene antagonists as add-on therapy in paediatric asthma. In my hands, the use of low-dose theophylline for an anti-inflammatory effect has been uniformly disappointing.

DIFFICULT EXERCISE-INDUCED ASTHMA

Exercise-induced asthma can be a real challenge in children, especially those with major sporting ambitions, who often only get asthma at the climax of a sporting occasion, when they least want it. If conventional use of short-acting β_2-agonists fails, choices include (alone or in combination): the use of long-acting β_2-agonists in the highest dose tolerated, or leukotriene receptor antagonists on the day of a sporting event; or the use of sodium cromoglycate or nedocromil prior to exercise. One oarsman whom I treat has found that nedocromil used every 30 min for 2½ hours before a race gives him total protection. These children are usually highly motivated and will try quite complex regimes. It is essential to emphasize that any medication must be checked to ensure that it is not on the banned substance list. Curing exercise-induced asthma by getting the athlete a doping ban is not popular.

Severe exercise-induced asthma must also be distinguished from a lack of cardiorespiratory fitness and psychological dyspnoea (below); neither are uncommon in high-performance, highly pressurized athletes.

GROWTH ISSUES

Any child treated for any chronic disease should have their height measured regularly and plotted on a growth chart. Sophisticated equipment and prolonged training are not necessary to get reasonably reproducible results. Any child with asthma, whatever the treatment, should have growth measured as part of the routine assessment. A thorough knowledge of normal growth is necessary in order to be able to interpret the abnormal. Atopic children, whether or not they have asthma and whether or not it is treated with inhaled corticosteroids, often show delay in puberty and a late growth spurt. This must not be mistaken for disease. Causes of growth delay in asthmatic children are listed in Box 7.5, of which much the most important is undertreated asthma. Properly used, inhaled steroids rarely cause growth delay. It is wise to use a large-volume spacer for their delivery if possible, and mouth rinsing after taking the medication should be advised. The lowest dose to control

---

- Physiological – prepubertal deceleration of growth with late-onset puberty.
- Undertreated asthma.
- Inhaled steroid therapy (particularly if overtreated, or also being treated with steroid nosedrops or skin creams).
- Coincidental disease – growth hormone deficiency, etc.

Box 7.5
The possible causes of growth suppression in children with asthma

symptoms should be prescribed. There is compelling evidence that overtreatment with inhaled steroids does cause growth suppression.

DRUG-DELIVERY DEVICES

The age-related choice of drug-delivery devices is given in Table 7.1. My own practice is based on the (possibly naïve) belief that if an older child is given a choice of drug-delivery devices, he or she is more likely actually to use it; compared with the minor differences between the various inhaled steroids and bronchodilators, the differences between devices in terms of aesthetic appeal are far more major. I usually send the child to the respiratory nurse to go through the available technology, and prescribe what he or she chooses, provided the child can use it. Importantly, spacers are seen as babyish, and metered dose inhalers as 'adult' and 'cool'; hence if inhaled steroids are prescribed in a spacer, inevitably the spacer will not be used. Although in theory the spacer is better than a dry-powder device, this is one example where excellent theory should give way to pragmatism.

Table 7.1
Age-related use of drug-delivery devices

Age (years)	Ideal device	Acceptable alternative
0–2	MDI + mask and spacer	Nebulizer[a]
3–6	MDI + spacer	Nebulizer[a]
6–12 (rescue therapy)	MDI + spacer, DPI, breath-activated inhaler	
6–12 (inhaled steroids)	MDI + spacer	DPI, breath-activated inhaler[b]
>12 (rescue therapy)	DPI, breath-activated inhaler[c]	
>12 (inhaled steroids)	MDI + spacer[d]	DPI, breath-activated inhaler
Acute exacerbation (all ages)	MDI + spacer	Nebulizer[e]

[a] Nebulizers must be used with a firmly attached face mask; they rarely if ever offer an advantage over the spacer and mask.
[b] Spacers are preferable, but some mothers cannot be dissuaded from discarding them; in such cases, a breath-activated device or DPD is preferable to MDI alone.
[c] I offer the choice of device to the adolescent, in the hope that adherence will be improved.
[d] The preferred option; inevitably the adolescent regards the spacer as 'babyish' and discards it, so another device must be used.
[e] For all but the most severe attacks, equivalent doses of rescue medication are equally effective by spacer and by nebulizer.
MDI, metered dose inhaler; DPI, dry-powder inhaler.

PSYCHOLOGY

The interactions between the brain and the airway are complex and fascinating. Ignorance of the psychology of asthma is a sure recipe for treatment failure. The combination of asthma and non-asthmatic respiratory symptoms is one of the most difficult situations of all.

Adherence

Complete adherence to all aspects of treatment is pathological. However, doctors probably consistently overestimate the degree of compliance, and in general are no more than 50 per cent accurate in estimating the degree of compliance in an individual child. One of the most common causes of difficult asthma is failure to take treatment. In one survey of computerized prescribing databases, only one child in six received enough prescriptions to cover asthma prophylaxis, even assuming that all medication was collected from the pharmacy and actually taken. Studies with peak flow meters containing a microchip show that after about 2 weeks, half the data are fabricated. The reasons for poor adherence are many, and the subject complex and unsolved.

If non-adherence is suspected, it is worth trying to check exactly how many prescriptions have actually been given out. Measurement of theophylline levels, and cortisol and prednisolone, may also help determine whether or not these medications are actually being taken.

Vocal cord dysfunction

This presents as treatment-resistant asthma. The child may have one or both of inspiratory or expiratory noisy breathing, worse when being observed or examined, better when attention has passed, and, absolutely characteristically, disappearing during sleep. Auscultation over the trachea reveals that the source of the noise is the upper airway. Typically, there is a 'hidden gain'; often the child is being pushed at school, and is failing to handle this. It is more common in adolescent girls. Almost invariably, these children have been overtreated by paediatricians (reasonably enough) terrified by the spectre of acute severe asthma. Treatment is, in the first instance, with relaxation and control of breathing exercises from a physiotherapist, or help from a skilled speech therapist. If this fails, the help of a skilled clinical psychologist should be sought.

Habit/honk cough

This noise is unmistakable. The cough is enormously loud, frequently repeated, invariant in character, hugely irritating to everyone who endures it for even the shortest time period, and quite unlike any organic cough. As with all the non-organic respiratory syndromes, the symptom disappears completely during sleep. Usually such children will have been treated with antibiotics and oral and inhaled steroids in escalating doses, because noise is thought to be directly proportional to the seriousness of the diagnosis. Treatment is along the line of vocal cord dysfunction (see above).

Hyperventilation syndromes

These are surprisingly common. It is always important to ask specific questions about perioral paraesthesiae and hand cramps during attacks. Sometimes the child will have identified an element of a panic attack, and that stress is a factor in asthma; if not, sensitive questions should be asked. These attacks may sometimes appear to respond to β_2-agonists, but typically take many activations, with the drug being used more for its effect as a psychological prop rather than for effects on airway receptors. Occasional children will use their rescue therapy very frequently, almost as a nervous tic. A further cause for repeated use of a metered dose inhaler is as a substance of abuse, using the propellant to get a 'high'.

Dealing with non-organic respiratory symptoms

It is pivotal that the child realizes that his account of his symptoms is accepted as genuine and accurate; that he is not making things up; and that he is not panicking or crazy. The approach must be that the symptoms are genuine and distressing, but are not due to asthma and will not respond to asthma treatment. Only then can an explanation of mechanisms be given, and appropriate interventions (as described above) initiated. It is usually not fruitful to try to dissect out the relative contributions of asthma, 'stress' and non-organic symptoms; any that are present should be treated appropriately.

REALLY DIFFICULT ASTHMA

Although most children with asthma respond well to inhaled steroids and long-acting bronchodilators, a few have recalcitrant symptoms. A checklist of important questions is given in Box 7.6. It is increasingly clear that not all difficult asthma is due to eosinophilic inflammation; the neutrophil may be important, and even non-inflammatory mechanisms. If the factors listed in Box 7.6 have been addressed, consideration should be given to referral for a

Box 7.6
Checklist of questions in the approach to the child with difficult asthma

- Does the child have asthma at all?
- Is the child taking the treatment (non-adherence, drug device not age-appropriate, complex regime)?
- Are there important environmental factors?
- Are there important psychological factors?
- Should the pathological phenotype be determined?

detailed evaluation, including measurement of inflammation using indirect (exhaled gas, induced sputum) and direct (bronchoalveolar lavage and endo-bronchial biopsy) methods, and determination of steroid receptor function. However, these investigations are only available in a few centres. None the less, it would seem a preferable approach to trying, at random, an ever-increasing cocktail of medications. For example, a symptomatic asthmatic, with marked bronchial hyperreactivity, but no evidence of inflammation, may benefit from continuous subcutaneous terbutaline infusions, whereas the child with eosinophilic bronchial inflammation, despite high-dose steroids, might be tried on cyclosporin. Much more work is needed, however, on the molecular and cellular phenotypes of difficult asthma, and how best to evaluate them clinically.

Summary

Childhood asthma comes in many different variants, not all inflammatory. There are unique aspects to almost all facets of management. Children, even those over age five years, are very different from miniature adults and should be treated differently. It is sad that such a common disease is not treated in an evidence-based fashion, because there is so little real evidence.

Current and future challenge of asthma

The past two decades have witnessed many important advances, both in terms of our understanding of the pathophysiology and of the management of asthma. The increasing information on epidemiology and natural history of asthma has led to many hypotheses that need testing, and that may lead ultimately to a better understanding of how asthma is triggered and why it is increasing in prevalence. The clinical importance of inflammatory processes in causing the symptoms of asthma has been realized, but the delineation of the exact processes in specific patients has not been achieved. Nevertheless the established treatment of asthma relies on targeting both the inflammatory process and on the relief of airways obstruction with bronchodilators. In terms of management, it is preferable to consider the two processes separately, each needing optimal control. This two-pronged approach will remain the basis of asthma therapy for a long time to come. Indeed, one of the recent advances in the treatment of moderately severe asthma is the use of combination therapy of a topical corticosteroid and a long-acting β-agonist.

The establishment of national and international guidelines has been instrumental in improving the care of the asthmatic, both through better education of the practitioner, as well as the asthmatic, and through implementation of the guidelines. Despite these improvements in knowledge and in treatments, there are still many unmet needs in asthma that need to be addressed.

Unmet needs in asthma

Estimates of the burden of asthma over the past few years indicate that there is a continuing problem. The Asthma Insights and Reality in Europe (AIRE) study, a telephone survey in seven European countries carried out in the spring of 1999, found that 38 per cent of children and 16 per cent of adults in the UK had lost school or work days due to their asthma in the past year. The AIRE study found that the household prevalence of diagnosed asthma was highest in the UK (15.2 per cent) and lowest in Germany (2.5 per cent). In the AIRE study, 27 per cent of asthma patients in the UK had required acute healthcare services over the preceding year. In 1999/2000, the National

Asthma campaign conducted a survey of a sample of 785 asthmatics and found that 20.9 per cent, 20.9 per cent and 41.7 per cent described their asthma as severe, moderate and mild, respectively, with 15.8 per cent stating that the asthma affected them quite a lot or a great deal. Nocturnal symptoms every night were found in 18 per cent, 16 per cent and 8 per cent of patients at Steps 5, 3 and 4, and 2 of the British management guidelines. In addition to persistent symptoms and severity, the number of asthma deaths persists, and the prevalence of asthma remains high and increasing. Clearly, there is a large unmet need in the asthmatic population, with persisting morbidity and mortality.

There are many potential reasons for the continuing burden of asthma. First, are patients receiving or taking adequate medication for their asthma? Unmet clinical needs in this area are summarized in Box 8.1. Are we giving treatment to the patients who really need it, and is there undertreatment with preventive therapy? There is evidence that many patients with asthma are undertreated, even in well-developed countries. Undertreatment may be due to inadequate evaluation and diagnosis, or problems with healthcare delivery, such as poor medical facilities in inner-city areas. Education of healthcare providers on asthma, and provision of care are important. From the point of view of the patient, there may be poor adherence to therapy – compliance to inhaled corticosteroid therapy has been reported to be between 30 and 50 per cent only. Poor compliance may result from many factors, such as fear of side-effects or poor doctor–patient relationship. Patients have to be taught how to use their inhalers and certain groups of patients have great difficulties with inhaled therapy, especially infants, the elderly and the disabled.

There are patients who are receiving preventative or prophylactic therapy, but not achieving adequate control of their asthma. These patients need review of their medications (perhaps increasing or adding therapies), environment and lifestyle. However, such reviews and change of therapies may be

Box 8.1
Unmet needs in asthma

- Improving adherence to treatments
- Delivery of asthma care
- Education of patients and self-management plans
- Implementation of asthma guidelines
- Prevention of asthma exacerbations
- Drug delivery systems
- Difficult-to-control asthma
- Irreversible airflow obstruction
- Asthma deaths

inadequate to achieve total symptom control. In such patients, one should ask whether their disease has a 'fixed' component that cannot be reversed by current therapies, or whether their disease is refractory to current therapies. There is some limited evidence that early intervention with anti-inflammatory treatment (usually inhaled corticosteroid therapy) may lead to a greater improvement in lung function. Delay in diagnosis and institution of preventive therapy may be associated with a lesser response. Alternatively, current therapies may not be efficacious in all patients with asthma, and there is a need for research and development of alternative therapies. Within this context, research is also needed to understand why the prevalence is increasing, in order that preventive measures can be taken.

Severe therapy-resistant asthma

Severe therapy-resistant asthma (or difficult-to-treat asthma) is poorly controlled asthma in terms of chronic symptoms, episodic exacerbations, persistent and variable airflow obstruction and a continued requirement for short-acting β-agonists, despite the use of high-dose inhaled corticosteroids, and often in addition to oral corticosteroid therapy. Therefore, these patients continue to experience persistent asthma despite taking maximum asthma therapies. Other terms that have been used to describe these patients include refractory asthma, steroid-dependent asthma, steroid-resistant asthma, difficult-to-control asthma, symptomatic asthma, life-threatening asthma and fatal asthma. Some of these terms indicate that there may be some resistance to the effects of anti-asthma treatments, particularly corticosteroids, in these patients. One of the major concerns of these patients is that they are exposed to the side-effects of high-dose inhaled and oral corticosteroid therapy; in addition, these patients have high level of morbidity and deterioration of quality of life, and an increased risk of dying of asthma.

The prevalence of severe therapy-resistant asthma is not known, but may represent 1–5 per cent of the asthmatic population, depending on the definition of severe asthma. However, this minority of patients may account for much of asthma costs, including medication, use of emergency rooms, hospitalization and death. It has been estimated that 80 per cent of asthma expenditure is consumed by only 20 per cent of the asthmatic population, who experience more severe disease. An average cost for each patient with severe asthma is nearly six times the cost of care for a patient with mild asthma.

The diagnosis of asthma rests on the clinical history and on physiological evidence of variable and reversible airflow obstruction. In the situation of severe therapy-resistant asthma, it is important to exclude other diseases that may masquerade as asthma (Box 2.3) and psychosocial factors. The patient should have been established on adequate doses of anti-asthma medication and it should be ascertained that the patient is adherent to the asthma therapies prescribed. Exacerbating factors for asthma, such as gastro-oesophageal reflux, rhinosinusitis, taking asthma-inducing drugs such as aspirin and β-blockers, and psychosocial factors, must be addressed and controlled. An approach to the evaluation of the patient with severe asthma is shown in Box 3.1.

There are different clinical patterns of severe therapy-resistant asthma, such as brittle asthma, chronic difficult asthma, fatal asthma and premenstrual worsening of asthma. This in itself would indicate that there may be different mechanisms involved in severe asthma. Brittle asthma was a term first used to describe patients with asthma who had a wide and chaotic variation in peak expiratory flow rate despite high doses of inhaled steroids, distinct from the controlled patterns of peak flow variation seen in 'usual' asthma. These patients have more life-threatening asthma because of the rapidity of onset of their severe attacks. This condition appears not to be controlled by inhaled or oral corticosteroid therapy, and may be helped by using high doses of β-adrenergic agonists, particularly administered subcutaneously. Some of these severe attacks may merge into near-fatal asthma episodes or fatal episodes. Impaired perception of airway narrowing and a reduced ventilatory response to hypoxia in some of these patients has been reported. In the fatality-prone asthmatic, retrospective analysis indicates that these patients are characterized by respiratory failure needing intubation, respiratory acidosis associated with an asthma attack not needing intubation, two or more hospitalizations for asthma despite the use of chronic oral corticosteroid therapy, and episodes of pneumomediastinum or pneumothorax associated with an attack of asthma. The risk of asthma death is also greater in those with previous attacks that occurred suddenly ('brittle' asthma) or were associated with hypoxic seizures, hypercapnia, very low peak flows and the use of medication from three or more classes of drugs for asthma.

The term 'chronic difficult asthma' is often used for patients affected by chronic symptoms interfering with sleep, exercise tolerance and the ability to work or attend school. There may be frequent exacerbations of these symptoms, which persist despite use of adequate asthma therapy. There may be evidence of reduced airflow limitation, and usually significant diurnal variation of peak flow. Higher doses of oral corticosteroids may lead to improvement in the control of asthma and airflow obstruction, but with corticosteroid dose reduction, control of asthma is lost. In these patients, the term corticosteroid-dependent asthma is used. Rarely, some patients with asthma demonstrate no symptomatic or physiological improvement with a course of oral corticosteroids (e.g. 40 mg of prednisolone per day for 2 weeks). These are 'corticosteroid-resistant' asthmatics.

The pathophysiology of chronic severe asthma is likely to be heterogeneous. Some studies indicate that there is greater degree of eosinophil activation in the airways, and that some patients show an excess of neutrophils. The extent to which the more distal airways are affected by the airway inflammatory process may also be important in determining severity. The airway hyper-responsiveness and the excessive airway narrowing may be the result of some intrinsic abnormality of the airway smooth muscle and of changes in the airway–parenchymal interactions. Finally, the loss of corticosteroid responsiveness may underlie all cases of severe asthma, and the causes may also be more than one, such as a reduction in binding affinity of the corticosteroid receptor and diminished binding to transcription factors of the activated corticosteroid receptor.

The management of patients with chronic severe asthma should ideally be undertaken in a centre with interest in asthma. A proper diagnostic and management evaluation may take 6–12 months to complete. Often, such patients may be taking unnecessarily high doses of inhaled or oral corticosteroids, which could be tapered to more acceptable levels. This often needs to be done in hospital because the patient may not be confident that dose-tapering is possible in his or her case. Addition of other therapies, such as long-acting β-agonists, slow-release theophylline and leukotriene inhibitors, are all worth trying, one at a time. The major aim of management is to reduce the need for a high dose of oral corticosteroids, since these are the most toxic drugs used by the severe asthmatic. Potentially toxic immunosuppressive agents, such as methotrexate (10–15 mg once per week), cyclosporin A (3 mg/kg per day) or auranofin (3 mg twice daily), a gold salt, may be tried as oral corticosteroid-sparing agents, as demonstrated in placebo-controlled double-blind randomized clinical trials. Usually, a treatment period of at least 3 months is necessary if any positive effect is to be observed. The average reduction in oral corticosteroid dosage achieved without reducing asthma control is of the order of 50 per cent. However, in clinical practice, these drugs have been disappointing, possibly because there is a large placebo effect. Immunoglobulin infusions have been reported to have a beneficial effect, but there have been no placebo-controlled trials. Patients taking high levels of oral corticosteroids should have bone densitometry measurements on a yearly basis and preventive measures against corticosteroid-induced osteoporosis should be instituted.

New approaches to the treatment of asthma

Although the current treatments for asthma are effective, there is a need for even more effective therapies targeted towards airway inflammatory processes, and towards bronchodilating the airways; in addition, it is likely that treatments aimed at 'airway wall remodelling' processes are needed. The development of new therapies has gathered pace. Over the past decade, more potent inhaled corticosteroids with less potential for systemic side-effects, and β-adrenergic agonist bronchodilators with a long duration of action, have been, and continue to be, developed. In addition, a new long-acting anti-cholinergic inhaler with a duration of effect of more than 24 hours has been developed. Although there are further efforts to improve these mainstay classes of drugs, it is unlikely that additional therapeutic gains will be large. Many specific targets have been identified in the inflammatory cascade of asthma. Leukotriene receptor antagonists were the first novel class of drugs introduced for the treatment of asthma over the past decade, and many more different classes will be tested over the next few years. Already, blocking certain mediators, such as the blocking of receptors of platelet-activating factor and of bradykinin, has not proven to be useful.

This era of novel potential therapies will be exciting, and will test whether inhibition of specific pathways in asthma is an effective therapeutic approach. This approach is usually aimed at inhibiting a specific pathway or molecule, although it is possible that more than one molecule or pathway may have to be inhibited for therapeutic success. Often, the efficacy of corticosteroids, drugs that work at several levels of the inflammatory process and suppress a whole range of cytokines and proteins, in controlling asthma is used to support the argument that inhibition of one pathway may not be successful in asthma. Nevertheless, new advances in molecular and cell biology have made it possible to develop specific monoclonal humanized antibodies and recombinant proteins, and also to inhibit transcription of specific genes by antisense technology.

The novel strategies that have been developed are shown in Box 8.2, and broadly involve the suppression of cytokines of the T-helper (Th) type 2 such as IL-4 and IL-5, using monoclonal antibodies or soluble recombinant

Box 8.2

New approaches to the therapy of asthma

1. Inhibition of the effects of IL-5 with anti-IL-5 monoclonal antibody.
2. Inhibition of the effects of IL-4 with soluble IL-4 receptor (IL-4Ra).
3. Promoting Th1 cytokines such as IFNγ or IL-12 in order to suppress the production and activity of Th2 cytokines.
4. Use anti-inflammatory cytokines such as IL-10 and IL-1Ra to inhibit asthmatic inflammation.
5. Inhibition of eosinophil migration and activation using an inhibitor of the adhesion molecule VLA-4 or ICAM-1, or using an antagonist to the chemokine receptor, CCR3.
6. Inhibition of IgE by using a monoclonal antibody to IgE (anti-IgE).

proteins to bind to and sequester bioactive cytokines; or the promotion or administration of T-helper type 1 cytokines such as IFNγ and IL-12, or of the anti-inflammatory cytokines such as IL-10 or IL-1Ra. Other Th2 cytokines that may be targeted include IL-9 and IL-13. Other strategies include inhibition of eosinophil migration or activation into airway tissues (such as receptor antagonists of the chemokine receptor, CCR3, or monoclonal antibodies or small molecule antagonists of the adhesion molecules ICAM-1 or VLA-4), or blocking the effect of IgE (such as using a monoclonal anti-IgE). Blocking transcription factors needed to generate chemokines/cytokines or blocking the cellular pathways that signal cellular reactions stimulated by these cytokines/chemokines are other approaches.

ANTI-IL-4 AND ANTI-IL-5 THERAPIES

IL-4 induces polarization of the Th0 cell to the Th2 phenotype, as well as isotype switch from IgM to IgE synthesis by B cells. In addition, it upregulates IgE receptors and VCAM-1 expression on vascular endothelium, thereby facilitating endothelial passage and accumulation of eosinophils and basophils. A recombinant soluble IL-4 receptor, which acts as an effective IL-4 receptor blocker, improves lung function and quality-of-life scores, and reduces rescue β_2-agonist requirement in asthma. In a 3-month study, this treatment improved FEV_1, and prevented deterioration in symptoms that were experienced in the parallel placebo-treated group. There were no serious side-effects, and the treatment was well tolerated. However, further development of this approach has been dropped.

IL-5 promotes eosinophil mobilization and trafficking, their maturation and maintenance. Two humanized forms of anti-IL-5 antibody have been tried in asthma (SB-240563 and Sch 55700). In mild asthmatics, SB-240563 inhibited blood eosinophil counts, and the eosinophil increase in sputum following allergen challenge. However, the clinical expression of allergen response was not affected, namely the early and late responses, and the accompanying increase in bronchial responsiveness. Trials in patients with more severe asthma have not shown any clinical benefits. Since the presence (or absence) of eosinophils in the tissues was not checked in these studies, it is not certain whether tissue eosinophilia was suppressed, and therefore whether adequate dosing was observed. The real effectiveness of the anti-IL-5 approach has not been totally tested.

ANTI-IgE THERAPY

A current novel therapy that has undergone clinical trials is anti-IgE. Because inhibition of allergic reactions may be achieved by antagonizing the effects of IgE, a monoclonal antibody targeted against IgE, referred to as anti-IgE or omalizumab, has been developed as a treatment for allergic diseases such as allergic asthma and allergic rhinitis. Omalizumab is a murine antibody which has been humanized such that the IgE-binding regions are comprised of only 5 per cent of murine components. It binds to the FcεRI binding site of the human IgE molecule, so that IgE can no longer bind to inflammatory cells such as basophils and mast cells. Omalizumab cannot interact with IgE already bound on basophils and mast cells and is not anaphylactogenic. It binds solely to free circulating IgE, forming small immune complexes that are stable and do not activate complement. Total serum IgE levels rise after omalizumab administration, but free serum IgE levels fall rapidly to about 5 per cent of baseline or less. Omalizumab reduces the number of FcεRI receptors on the surface of basophils, and histamine release from basophils in response to house dust mite allergen. Thus, free IgE regulates the expression of FcεRI expression.

Clinical effects of omalizumab

Omalizumab decreases mean serum IgE levels by 98 per cent, and effectively attenuates allergen-induced early- and late-phase bronchoconstriction, and also methacholine bronchial hyperresponsiveness, with a reduction in the percentage of eosinophils in induced sputum and the number of circulating eosinophils. Several trials of omalizumab have now been performed in patients with moderate to severe allergic asthma, both adults and children. In a recent randomized, double-blind, placebo-controlled trial in 317 patients with moderate to severe allergic asthma requiring inhaled and/or oral corticosteroids, the patients received either placebo, omalizumab 2.5 μg/kg per monogram of IgE per ml (low dose) or omalizumab 5.8 μg/kg per monogram of IgE per ml (high dose), intravenously on days 0 (half a dose), 4 (half a dose) and 7 (full dose) and then at biweekly intervals for 20 weeks. During the last 8 weeks of treatment, the corticosteroid dosages were tapered. Both high- and low-dose omalizumab produced a greater than 95 per cent mean decrease in serum IgE levels. A higher proportion of patients in the high-dose and low-dose omalizumab groups experienced a 50 per cent reduction in asthma symptom scores than in the placebo group. Similarly, there was a significantly higher proportion of patients in the high-dose group than in the low-dose group and placebo groups who were able to achieve a 50 per cent of reduction in oral corticosteroids. In the high-dose, low-dose and placebo groups, respectively, oral corticosteroids were stopped in 33, 43 and 17 per cent of patients, and inhaled steroids in 18, 23 and 12 per cent of patients. Compared to placebo, the improvement in mean morning peak expiratory flow from baseline to week 12 was significantly greater in the high-dose group (+30.7 L/min; $P = 0.007$), but not in the low-dose group (+18.6 L/min). Rescue β-agonist use and the proportion of patients experiencing asthma exacerbations were lower in the group treated with omalizumab. There were no significant differences in adverse events between actively treated and placebo group, with no reports of serious drug-related adverse events.

Two double-blind, randomized, parallel group, placebo-controlled studies have recently been presented, involving 1071 patients (adolescents and adults) with moderate to severe allergic asthmatic treated with subcutaneous omalizumab. Overall, the percentage of patients having at least one exacerbation was nearly twice a high in the placebo group as in the omalizumab groups. Daytime and nocturnal asthma symptoms and FEV_1 significantly improved with omalizumab compared to placebo. During the steroid withdrawal phase, more than twice as many patients in the omalizumab group as in the placebo group discontinued inhaled corticosteroid completely. The omalizumab group used significantly less rescue β_2-agonist. Similar results have been reported in children, where there was a lower number of exacerbations and a reduced need for β_2-agonist rescue medication in the omalizumab group. More subjects in the omalizumab group decreased their dose of inhaled corticosteroids, with complete withdrawal in 55 per cent of the omalizumab group versus 39 per cent in the placebo group. A reduction in symptoms of rhinitis and in antihistamine use has been reported in patients with seasonal birch-pollen rhinitis when treated with omalizumab.

Omalizumab appears to be a safe and effective treatment of moderate to severe allergic asthma, offering the potential for discontinuing or decreasing corticosteriod use associated with an improved control of asthma and with a reduction in the incidence of asthma exacerbations in children and adults. Omalizumab has not been compared to other add-on therapies which have also demonstrated additive effects to inhaled corticosteroids in improving lung function and reducing the incidence of exacerbations (e.g. long-acting β-agonist and leukotriene inhibitors). Because the mechanism of action of omalizumab is different from that of other existing anti-asthma medication, it is possible that its clinical effects may be additive to the effects of these medications. Omalizumab offers the following advantages for patients with moderate to severe allergic asthma:

1. targeting the allergic component of asthma directly for the first time;
2. concomitant treatment of associated allergic diseases such as rhinitis and eczema;
3. reducing the dose of inhaled or oral corticosteroids, therefore the risks of adverse events from steroids;
4. the opportunity to control adherence to therapy, since the injections (once- or twice-monthly subcutaneous injections) are to be delivered by a nurse.

Monoclonal antibody treatment in asthma is a new approach and the pharmaco-economic factors are not worked out yet. Production of omalizumab is expensive, as for other monoclonal antibodies, but omalizumab can be justified in patients with more severe asthma on high-dose inhaled steroids and with exacerbations needing frequent acute and chronic medical attention. Omalizumab is the only drug with a new mechanism of action likely to be licensed for treatment of allergic asthma in the near future, and may be particularly useful in the treatment of severe asthma.

The concept of disease remission

Disease remission in asthma is a new concept that should be discussed since, amongst the new agents that may become available for the treatment of asthma (Box 8.1), there may be medicines that could prevent the further progression of the disease process. The concept is that a drug administered over a short period of time leads to a disappearance of the disease (symptoms, exacerbations and possibly an aspect of the inflammatory process) over a prolonged period of time, usually more than 3 months. Inhaled corticosteroids may fall in this category, since stopping treatment with inhaled steroids may be associated with a variable time lag before symptoms recur (weeks to months). Mechanistically, it is not clear whether this process of disease remission in asthma is related to preventing (or reversing) further structural remodelling. Such a concept needs to be defined so that appropriate clinical trials can be carried out with this in mind. It is too early to discuss a cure, but this may be the first step in the right direction.

Towards prevention of allergies and asthma

It is evident that one of the most effective ways of tackling the problem of asthma is to take preventive measures for such a common disease. Because asthma is mostly associated with allergies, prevention of allergies may lead to prevention of asthma. Many hypotheses regarding the development of allergies and asthma are currently being tested, and such studies may pinpoint the exact risk factors and the immunological mechanisms that lead to the development of allergies and asthma. For some years now, an imbalance of the Th1 and Th2 immune responses towards the Th2 has held forth as being the fundamental immunological defect. An indirect way of modulating Th1/Th2 balance has been to boost innate immunity by the use of vaccines, particularly for the redirection of the Th2 response in favour of the Th1 response. This concept was first supported by a study in Japanese schoolchildren, in whom an association between BCG vaccination and a diminished incidence of atopy and allergic disease was observed. This suggested a role for early mycobacterial exposure in the development of atopic responsiveness, which would induce a strong Th1 immune response. The beneficial effects of specific immunotherapy may result from increasing Th1 immune responses, and the development of immunotherapy using peptide sequences of allergens (e.g. cat allergens) may lead to more effective and safer treatment for specific allergies. Several other approaches to alter the Th2/Th1 balance are being investigated, including the use of the bacterial immunostimulator, CpG, raising the possibility of prevention of the development of asthma and allergic diseases. However, it has to be said that there are several drawbacks to this approach, of which the greatest concern is that a Th1 exuberance may lead to other autoimmune diseases, such as multiple sclerosis or rheumatoid arthritis.

Responders and non-responders: pharmacogenomics

One of the recent findings regarding therapeutic responses to asthma treatments is that a substantial proportion of the individual therapeutic responses to treatment are genetically determined. The two best examples of genetically determined therapeutic responses related to asthma therapy include responses to β-adrenergic agonists and leukotriene inhibitors. Nine polymorphisms have been described in the β_2-adrenoceptor gene, of which four result in single amino-acid substitutions. The glycine substitution for arginine at amino acid 16 (Gly16) has been associated with more severe asthma, and with a greater propensity for bronchodilator desensitization after the regular use of formoterol. Patients who were homozygous for Arg16 had increased bronchial responsiveness to metacholine, compared with their responsiveness when they did not receive regular treatment with a β-agonist, fenoterol.

A family of polymorphisms exists in the promoter of the gene for 5-lipoxygenase (ALOX5) enzyme, which is crucial in the generation of cysteinyl-leukotrienes. A polymorphism of the ALOX5 promoter displays less capacity for gene transcription than the wild-type ALOX5 promoter, and therefore could underlie therapeutic responses to inhibitors of 5-lipoxgenase enzymes. The improvement in FEV_1 observed with treatment of mild to moderate asthmatics with leukotriene inhibitors is variable. In a study with an ALOX5 inhibitor, patients with wild-type ALOX5 promoter responded with a mean increase in FEV_1 of 18.8 per cent, while in patients with mutant-type ALOX5 promoter, the change in FEV_1 was negligible, at -1.1 per cent. It is likely that more than one genetic polymorphism may explain the overall therapeutic response to drugs, and use of pharmacogenomics may be useful for tailoring drugs to the individual asthmatic patients that will respond best, thus ensuring optimal targeting of drug therapy.

Conclusion

The past decade of research into asthma has given hope for both prevention and more effective treatments than currently available. For all new treatments, a considerable amount of time will be devoted to the assessment of their efficacy in clinical trials before they can be used widely for the treatment of (or for the prevention of) asthma. Although much more benefit than is currently derived can be obtained from implementation of asthma guidelines and from making sure that patients adhere to their treatments, it is clear that new forms of treatments are much needed, because not all patients with asthma respond adequately to currently available treatments.

Bibliography

Chapter 1

Anderson, H.R., Butland, B.K. and Strachan, D.P. (1994) Trends in prevalence and severity of childhood asthma. *BMJ* **308**, 1600–4.

Beasley, R., Pearce, N., Crane, J., Windorn, H. and Burgess, C. (1991) Asthma mortality and inhaled β-agonist therapy. *Aust. NZ J. Med.* **21**, 753–63.

Brand, P.L., Postma, D.S., Kerstjens, H.A. and Koeter, G.H. (1991) Relationship of airway hyperresponsiveness to respiratory symptoms and diurnal peak flow variation in patients with obstructive lung disease. The Dutch CNSLD Study Group. *Am. Rev. Respir. Dis.* **143**, 916–21.

Campbell, M.J., Cogman, G.R., Holgate, S.T. and Johnston, S.L. (1997) Age specific trends in asthma mortality in England and Wales, 1983–95: results of an observational study. *BMJ* **314**, 1439–41.

Ciba Guest Symposium (1959) Terminology, definition and classification of chronic pulmonary emphysema and related conditions. *Thorax* **14**, 286–99.

Cockcroft, D.W., Killian, D.N., Mellon, J.J.A. and Hargreave, F.E. (1977) Bronchial reactivity to inhaled histamine: a method and clinical survey. *Clin. Allergy* **7**, 235–43.

Djukanovic, R., Roche, W.R., Wilson, J.W. *et al.* (1990) Mucosal inflammation in asthma. *Am. Rev. Respir. Dis.* **142**, 434–57.

Finucane, K.E., Greville, H.W. and Brown, P.J. (1985) Irreversible airflow obstruction. Evolution in asthma. *Med. J. Aust.* **142**, 602–4.

Fletcher, C.M. and Pride, N.B. (1984) Definitions of emphysema, chronic bronchitis, asthma, and airflow obstruction: 25 years on from the Ciba symposium. *Thorax* **39**, 81–5.

International Study of Asthma and Allergies in Childhood (ISAAC) Steering Committee (1998) Worldwide variation in prevalence of symptoms of asthma, allergic rhinoconjunctivitis, and atopic eczema: ISAAC. *Lancet* **351**, 1225–32 [see comments].

Kaur, B., Anderson, H.R., Austin, J. *et al.* (1998) Prevalence of asthma symptoms, diagnosis, and treatment in 12–14 year old children across Great Britain (International Study of Asthma and Allergies in Childhood, ISAAC UK). *BMJ* **316**, 118–24.

Lange, P., Parner, J., Vestbo, J., Schnohr, P. and Jensen, G. (1998) A 15-year follow-up study of ventilatory function in adults with asthma. *N. Engl. J. Med.* **339**, 1194–2000.

Martinez, F.D., Wright, A.L., Taussig, L.M., Holberg, C.J., Halonen, M. and Morgan, W.J. (1995) Asthma and wheezing in the first six years of life. The Group Health Medical Associates. *N. Engl. J. Med.* **332**, 133–8.

National Asthma Campaign (1999) *National Asthma Audit 1999/2000*. Direct Publishing Ltd, Berkshire.

Ninan, T.K. and Russell, G. (1992) Respiratory symptoms and atopy in Aberdeen schoolchildren: evidence from two surveys 25 years apart. *BMJ* **304**, 873–5.

Panhuysen, C.I., Vonk, J.M., Koeter, G.H. *et al.* (1997) Adult patients may outgrow their asthma: a 25-year follow-up study. *Am. J. Respir. Crit. Care Med.* **155**, 1267–72.

Pattemore, P.K., Asher, M.I., Harrison, A.C., Mitchell, E.A., Rea, H.H. and Stewart, A.W. (1990) The interrelationship among bronchial hyperresponsiveness, the diagnosis of asthma, and asthma symptoms. *Am. Rev. Respir. Dis.* **142**, 549–54.

Rabe, K.F., Vermeire, P.A., Soriano, J.B. and Maier, W.C. (2000) Clinical management of asthma in 1999: the Asthma Insights and Reality in Europe (AIRE) study. *Eur. Respir. J.* **16**, 802–7.

Chapter 2

Ayres, J.G., Miles, J.F. and Barnes, P.J. (1998) Brittle asthma. *Thorax* **53**, 315–21.

Brightling, C.E., Monteiro, W., Ward, R. *et al.* (2000) Sputum eosinophilia and short-term response to prednisolone in chronic obstructive pulmonary disease: a randomised controlled trial. *Lancet* **356**, 1480–5.

Britton, J. (1998) Symptoms and objective measures to define the asthma phenotype. *Clin. Exp. Allergy* **28** (suppl. 1), 2–7.

Burney, P.G., Laitinen, L.A., Perdrizet, S. *et al.* (1989) Validity and repeatability of the IUATLD (1984) Bronchial Symptoms Questionnaire: an international comparison. *Eur. Respir. J.* **2**, 940–5.

Carrao, W.M., Braman, S.S. and Irwin, R.S. (1979) Chronic cough as the sole presenting manifestation of bronchial asthma. *N. Engl. J. Med.* **300**, 633–7.

Chanez, P., Vignola, A.M., O'Shaugnessy, T. *et al.* (1997) Corticosteroid reversibility in COPD is related to features of asthma. *Am. J. Respir. Crit. Care Med.* **155**, 1529–34.

Christopher, K.L., Wood, R.P., Eckert, R.C., Blager, F.B., Raney, R.A. and Souhrada, J.F. (1983) Vocal-cord dysfunction presenting as asthma. *N. Engl. J. Med.* **308**, 1566–70.

Gibson, P.G. (2000) Monitoring the patient with asthma: an evidence-based approach. *J. Allergy Clin. Immunol.* **106**, 17–26.

Kogevinas, M., Anto, J.M., Sunyer, J., Tobias, A., Kromhout, H. and Burney, P. (1999) Occupational asthma in Europe and other industrialised areas: a population-based study. European Community Respiratory Health Survey Study Group. *Lancet* **353**, 1750–4.

Martin, R.J. (1993) Nocturnal asthma: circadian rhythms and therapeutic interventions. *Am. Rev. Respir. Dis.* **147**, S25–8.

McFadden, E.R. Jr and Gilbert, I.A. (1994) Exercise-induced asthma. *N. Engl. J. Med.* **330**, 1362–7.

Reddel, H., Ware, S., Marks, G., Salome, C., Jenkins, C. and Woolcock, A. (1999) Differences between asthma exacerbations and poor asthma control. *Lancet* **353**, 364–9.

Redier, H., Daures, J.P., Michel, C. *et al.* (1995) Assessment of the severity of asthma by an expert system. Description and evaluation. *Am. J. Respir. Crit. Care Med.* **151**, 345–52.

Chapter 3

Boulet, L.P., Cartier, A., Thomson, N.C., Roberts, R.S., Dolovich, J. and Hargreave, F.E. (1983) Asthma and increases in nonallergic bronchial responsiveness from seasonal pollen exposure. *J. Allergy Clin. Immunol.* **71**, 399–406.

Burrows, B., Martinez, F.D. and Halonen, M. (1989) Association of asthma with serum IgE levels and skin-test reactivity to allergens. *N. Engl. J. Med.* **320**, 271–2.

Carr, D.H., Hibon, S., Rubens, M. and Chung, K.F. (1998) Peripheral airways obstruction on high-resolution computed tomography in chronic severe asthma. *Respir. Med.* **92**, 448–53.

Custovic, A., Simpson, A., Chapman, M.D. and Woodcock, A. (1998) Allergen avoidance in the treatment of asthma and atopic disorders. *Thorax* **53**, 63–72.

Gibson, P.G., Wong, B.J., Hepperle, M.J. *et al.* (1992) A research method to induce and examine a mild exacerbation of asthma by withdrawal of inhaled corticosteroid. *Clin. Exp. Allergy* **22**, 525–32.

Higgins, B.G., Britton, J.R., Chinn, S. *et al.* (1989) The distribution of peak expiratory flow variability in a population sample. *Am. Rev. Respir. Dis.* **140**, 1368–72.

Jayaram, L., Parameswaran, K., Sears, M.R. and Hargreave, F.E. (2000) Induced sputum cell counts: their usefulness in clinical practice. *Eur. Respir. J.* **16**, 150–8.

Jones, P.W., Quirk, F.H., Baveystock, C.M. and Littlejohns, P. (1992) A self-complete measure of health status for chronic airflow limitation. The St. George's Respiratory Questionnaire. *Am. Rev. Respir. Dis.* **145**, 1321–7.

Juniper, E.F., Buist, A.S., Cox, F.M., Ferrie, P.J. and King, D.R. (1999) Validation of a standardized version of the Asthma Quality of Life Questionnaire. *Chest* **115**, 1265–70.

Kharitonov, S., Alving, K. and Barnes, P.J. (1997) Exhaled and nasal nitric oxide measurements: recommendations. The European Respiratory Society Task Force. *Eur. Respir. J.* **10**, 1683–93.

Miller, M.R., Dickinson, S.A. and Hitchings, D.J. (1992) The accuracy of portable peak flow meters. *Thorax* **47**, 904–9.

Paganin, F., Trussard, V., Seneterre, E. *et al.* (1992) Chest radiography and high-resolution computed tomography of the lungs in asthma. *Am. Rev. Respir. Dis.* **146**, 1084–7.

Pizzichini, E., Pizzichini, M.M., Gibson, P. *et al.* (1998) Sputum eosinophilia predicts benefit from prednisone in smokers with chronic obstructive bronchitis. *Am. J. Respir. Crit. Care Med.* **158**, 1511–17.

Platts-Mills, T.A., Mitchell, E.B., Nock, P., Tovey, E.R., Moszar, H. and Wilkins, S. (1982) Reduction of bronchial hyperreactivity during prolonged allergen avoidance. *Lancet* **ii**, 675–8.

Woolcock, A.J., Salome, C.M. and Yan, K. (1984) The shape of the dose–response curve to histamine in asthmatic and normal subjects. *Am. Rev. Respir. Dis.* **130**, 71–5.

Zimmerman, B., Feanny, S., Reisman, J. *et al.* (1988) Allergy in asthma. I. The dose relationship of allergy to severity of childhood asthma. *J. Allergy Clin. Immunol.* **81**, 63–70.

Chapter 4

Barnes, P.J., Chung, K.F. and Page, C.P. (1998) Inflammatory mediators of asthma: an update. *Pharmacol. Rev.* **50**, 515–96.

Bousquet, J., Jeffery, P.K., Busse, W.W., Johnson, M. and Vignola, A.M. (2000) Asthma. From bronchoconstriction to airways inflammation and remodeling. *Am. J. Respir. Crit. Care Med.* **161**, 1720–45.

Busse, W.W., Banks-Schlegel, S. and Wenzel, S.E. (2000) Pathophysiology of severe asthma. *J. Allergy Clin. Immunol.* **106**, 1033–42.

Chung, K.F. (1986) Role played by inflammation in the hyperreactivity of the airways in asthma. *Thorax* **41**, 657–62.

Chung, K.F. (2000) Airway smooth muscle cells: contributing to and regulating airway mucosal inflammation? *Eur. Respir. J.* **15**, 961–8.

Chung, K.F. and Barnes, P.J. (1999) Cytokines in asthma. *Thorax* **54**, 825–57.

Cookson, W.O. and Moffatt, M.F. (2000) Genetics of asthma and allergic disease. *Hum. Mol. Genet.* **9**, 2359–64.

Holt, P.G. (2000) Antigen presentation in the lung. *Am. J. Respir. Crit. Care Med.* **162**, S151–6.

Holt, P.G. and Stumbles, P.A. (2000) Regulation of immunologic homeostasis in peripheral tissues by dendritic cells: the respiratory tract as a paradigm. *J. Allergy Clin. Immunol.* **105**, 421–9.

James, A.L., Pare, P.D. and Hogg, J.C. (1989) The mechanics of airway narrowing in asthma. *Am. Rev. Respir. Dis.* **139**, 242–6.

Johnston, S.L. (1995) Natural and experimental rhinovirus infections of the lower respiratory tract. *Am. J. Respir. Crit. Care Med.* **152**, S46–52.

Nickel, R., Beck, L.A., Stellato, C. and Schleimer, R.P. (1999) Chemokines and allergic disease. *J. Allergy Clin. Immunol.* **104**, 723–42.

Redington, A.E. and Howarth, P.H. (1997) Airway wall remodelling in asthma [editorial]. *Thorax* **52**, 310–12.

Romagnani, S. (2000) The role of lymphocytes in allergic disease. *J. Allergy Clin. Immunol.* **105**, 399–408.

Rothenberg, M.E. (1998) Eosinophilia. *N. Engl. J. Med.* **338**, 1592–1600.

Sandberg, S., Paton, J.Y., Ahola, S. *et al.* (2000) The role of acute and chronic stress in asthma attacks in children. *Lancet* **356**, 982–7.

Strachan, D.P. (1989) Hay fever, hygiene, and household size. *BMJ* **299**, 1259–60.

Strachan, D.P. and Cook, D.G. (1998) Health effects of passive smoking. 5. Parental smoking and allergic sensitisation in children. *Thorax* **53**, 117–23.

von Mutius, E., Martinez, F.D., Fritzsch, C., Nicolai, T., Roell, G. and Thiemann, H.H. (1994) Prevalence of asthma and atopy in two areas of West and East Germany. *Am. J. Respir. Crit. Care Med.* **149**, 358–64.

Chapter 5

Agertoft, L. and Pedersen, S. (2000) Effect of long-term treatment with inhaled budesonide on adult height in children with asthma. *N. Engl. J. Med.* **343**, 1064–9.

Altman, L.C., Munk, Z., Seltzer, J. *et al.* (1998) A placebo-controlled, dose-ranging study of montelukast, a cysteinyl leukotriene-receptor antagonist. Montelukast Asthma Study Group. *J. Allergy Clin. Immunol.* **102**, 50–6.

Barnes, P.J., Pedersen, S. and Busse, W.W. (1993) Efficacy and safety of inhaled corticosteroids in asthma: an update. *Am. J. Respir. Crit. Care Med.* **157**, S1–S53.

Bousquet, J., Lockey, R., Malling, H.J. *et al.* (1998) Allergen immunotherapy: therapeutic vaccines for allergic diseases. World Health Organization. American academy of Allergy, Asthma and Immunology. *Ann. Allergy Asthma Immunol.* **81**, 401–5.

Busse, W.W., Chervinsky, P., Condemi, J. *et al.* (1998) Budesonide delivered by Turbuhaler is effective in a dose-dependent fashion when used in the treatment of adult patients with chronic asthma. *J. Allergy Clin. Immunol.* **101**, 457–63.

Childhood Asthma Management Program Research Group (2000) Long-term effects of budesonide or nedocromil in children with asthma. *N. Engl. J. Med.* **343**, 1054–63.

Drazen, J.M., Israel, E., Boushey, H.A. *et al.* (1996) Comparison of regularly scheduled with as-needed use of albuterol in mild asthma. Asthma Clinical Research Network. *N. Engl. J. Med.* **335**, 841–7 [see comments].

Drazen, J.M., Israel, E. and O'Byrne, P.M. (1999) Treatment of asthma with drugs modifying the leukotriene pathway. *N. Engl. J. Med.* **340**, 197–206.

Durham, S.R., Walker, S.M., Varga, E.M. *et al.* (1999) Long-term clinical efficacy of grass-pollen immunotherapy. *N. Engl. J. Med.* **341**, 468–75.

Evans, D.J., Taylor, D.A., Zetterstrom, O., Chung, K.F., O'Connor, B.J. and Barnes, P.J. (1997) A comparison of low-dose inhaled budesonide plus theophylline and high-dose inhaled budesonide for moderate asthma. *N. Engl. J. Med.* **337**, 1412–18 [see comments].

Fish, J.E., Karpel, J.P., Craig, T.J. *et al.* (2000) Inhaled mometasone furoate reduces oral prednisone requirements while improving respiratory function and health-related quality of life in patients with severe persistent asthma. *J. Allergy Clin. Immunol.* **106**, 852–60.

Greening, A.P., Ind, P.W., Northfield, M. and Shaw, G. (1994) Added salmeterol versus higher-dose corticosteroid in asthma patients with symptoms on existing inhaled corticosteroid. *Lancet* **344**, 219–24.

Haahtela, T., Jarvinen, M., Kava, T. *et al.* (1991) Comparison of a β_2-agonist, terbutaline, with an inhaled corticosteroid, budesonide, in newly detected asthma. *N. Engl. J. Med.* **325**, 388–92.

Haahtela, T., Jarvinen, M., Kava, T. *et al.* (1994) Effects of reducing or discontinuing inhaled budesonide in patients with mild asthma. *N. Engl. J. Med.* **331**, 700–5 [see comments].

International Study of Asthma and Allergies in Childhood (ISAAC) Steering Committee (1998) Worldwide variation in prevalence of symptoms of asthma, allergic rhinoconjunctivitis, and atopic eczema: ISAAC. *Lancet* **351**, 1225–32.

Kemp, J.P., Berkowitz, R.B., Miller, S.D., Murray, J.J., Nolop, K. and Harrison, J.E. Mometasone furoate administered once daily is as effective as twice-daily administration for treatment of mild-to-moderate persistent asthma. *J. Allergy Clin. Immunol.* **106**, 485–92.

Lipworth, B.J. (1995) New perspectives on inhaled drug delivery and systemic bioactivity. *Thorax* **50**, 105–10.

Lofdahl, C.G., Reiss, T.F., Leff, J.A. *et al.* (1999) Randomised, placebo controlled trial of effect of a leukotriene receptor antagonist, montelukast, on tapering inhaled corticosteroids in asthmatic patients. *BMJ* **319**, 87–90.

Nelson, H.S. (1995) Beta-adrenergic bronchodilators. *N. Engl. J. Med.* **333**, 499–506.

Nelson, H.S., Busse, W.W., deBoisblanc, B.P. *et al.* (1999) Fluticasone propionate powder: oral corticosteroid-sparing effect and improved lung function and quality of life in patients with severe chronic asthma. *J. Allergy Clin. Immunol.* **103**, 267–75.

Noonan, M., Chervinsky, P., Busse, W.W. *et al.* (1995) Fluticasone propionate reduces oral prednisone use while it improves asthma control and quality of life. *Am. J. Respir. Crit. Care Med.* **152**, 1467–73.

O'Callaghan, C. and Barry, P.W. (2000) How to choose delivery devices for asthma. *Arch. Dis. Child.* **82**, 185–7.

Pauwels, R.A., Lofdahl, C., Postma, D. *et al.* (1997) Effect of inhaled formoterol and budesonide on exacerbations of asthma. *N. Engl. J. Med.* **337**, 1405–11.

Pearlman, D.S., Chervinsky, P., Laforce, C. *et al.* (1992) A comparison of salmeterol with albuterol in the treatment of mild-to-moderate asthma. *N. Engl. J. Med.* **327**, 1420–5.

Schuh, S., Reisman, J., Alshehri, M. *et al.* (2000) A comparison of inhaled fluticasone and oral prednisone for children with severe acute asthma. *N. Engl. J. Med.* **343**, 689–94.

Spector, S.L., Smith, L.J. and Glass, M. (1994) Effects of 6 weeks of therapy with oral doses of ICI 204, 219, a leukotriene D_4 receptor antagonists, in subjects with bronchial asthma. *Am. J. Resp. Crit. Care Med.* **150**, 618–32.

Stirling, R.G. and Chung, K.F. (2000) New immunological approaches and cytokine targets in asthma and allergy. *Eur. Respir. J.* **16**, 1158–74.

Weinberger, M. and Hendeles, L. (1996) Theophylline in asthma. *N. Engl. J. Med.* **334**, 1380–8.

Chapter 6

Anto, J.M., Sunyer, J., Reed, C.E. *et al.* (1993) Preventing asthma epidemics due to soybeans by dust-control measures. *N. Engl. J. Med.* **329**, 1760–3.

Barr, R.G., Woodruff, P.G., Clark, S. and Camargo, C.A. Jr (2000) Sudden-onset asthma exacerbations: clinical features, response to therapy, and 2-week follow-up. Multicenter Airway Research Collaboration (MARC) investigators. *Eur. Respir. J.* **15**, 266–73.

Boulet, L.P., Becker, A., Berube, D. *et al.* (1999) Canadian asthma consensus report. *Can. Med. Assoc. J.* **161**, S1–61.

British Thoracic Society (1993) Guidelines on the management of asthma. *Thorax* **48** (suppl.), S1–24.

British Thoracic Society (1997) The British guidelines on asthma management 1995. Review and position statement. *Thorax* **52** (suppl. 1).

Charlton, I., Charlton, G., Broomfield, J. and Mullee, M.A. (1990) Evaluation of peak flow and symptoms only self management plans for control of asthma in general practice. *BMJ* **301**, 1355–9.

D'Souza, W., Burgess, C., Ayson, M., Crane, J., Pearce, N. and Beasley, R. (1996) Trial of a 'credit card' asthma self-management plan in a high-risk group of patients with asthma. *J. Allergy Clin. Immunol.* **97**, 1085–92.

Gibson, P.G., Coughlan, J., Wilson, A.J. *et al.* (2000) Self-management education and regular practitioner review for adults with asthma. *Cochrane Database Syst. Rev.* CD001117.

Global Initiative for Asthma (1995) Global strategy for asthma management and prevention. NHLBI/WHO Workshop Report. National Institutes of Health, National Heart Lung and Blood Institute.

Lahdensuo, A. (1999) Guided self management of asthma – how to do it. *BMJ* **319**, 759–60.

Partridge, M.R., Fabbri, L.M. and Chung, K.F. (2000) Delivering effective asthma care – how do we implement asthma guidelines? *Eur. Respir. J.* **15**, 235–7.

Rodrigo, G.J. and Rodrigo, C. (2000) Rapid-onset asthma attack: a prospective cohort study about characteristics and response to emergency department treatment. *Chest* **118**, 1547–52.

Salmeron, S., Liard, R., Eckharrat, D, Muir, J.F., Neukirch, F. and Ellrodt, A. (2001) Asthma severity and adequacy of management in emergency departments: a prospective study of 3772 cases. *Lancet* **358**, 629–35.

Stenius-Aarniala, B., Piirila, P. and Teramo, K. (1988) Asthma and pregnancy: a prospective study of 198 pregnancies. *Thorax* **43**, 12–18.

Woolcock, A., Rubinfeld, A.R., Seale, J.P. *et al.* (1989) Asthma Management Plan, 1989. *Med. J. Aust.* **151**, 650–2.

Chapter 7

Agertoft, L. and Pedersen, S. (1994) Effects of long-term treatment with an inhaled steroid on growth and lung function in asthmatic children. *Respir. Med.* **88**, 373–81.

Bisgaard, H. (2000) Long acting β_2 agonists in management of childhood asthma: a critical review of the literature. *Pediatr. Pulmonol.* **29**, 221–34.

Bjorkstein, F. and Suoniemi, I. (1981) Time and intensity of first pollen contacts and risk of subsequent pollen allergies. *Acta Med. Scand.* **209**, 299–303.

Cane, R.S. and McKenzie, S.A. (2001) Parents interpretation of children's respiratory symptoms on video. *Arch. Dis. Child.* **84**, 31–4.

Clarke, J.R., Reese, A. and Silverman, M. (1992) Bronchial responsiveness and lung function in infants with lower respiratory tract illness over the first six months of life. *Arch. Dis. Child.* **67**, 1454–8.

Elphick, H.E., Sherlock, P., Foxall, G. *et al.* (2001) Survey of respiratory sounds in infants. *Arch. Dis. Child.* **84**, 35–9.

Koh, Y.Y., Jeong, J.Y., Park, Y. and Kim, C.K. (1999) Development of wheezing in patients with cough variant asthma during an increase in airway responsiveness. *Eur. Respir. J.* **14**, 302–8.

Martinez, F.D., Morgan, W.J., Wright, A.L. *et al.* (1988) Diminished lung function as a predisposing factor for wheezing respiratory illness in infants. *N. Engl. J. Med.* **319**, 1112–17.

Oswald, H., Phelan, P.D., Lanigan, A., Hibbert, M., Bowes, G. and Olinsky, A. (1994) Outcome of childhood asthma in mid-adult life. *BMJ* **309**, 95–6.

Oswald, H., Phelan, P.D., Lanigan, A. *et al.* (1997) Childhood asthma and lung function in mid-adult life. *Pediatr. Pulmonol.* **23**, 14–20.

Redline, S., Wright, E.C., Kattan, M., Kercsmar, C. and Weiss, K. (1996) Short term compliance with peak flow monitoring: results from a study of inner city children with asthma. *Pediatr. Pulmonol.* **21**, 203–10.

Strachan, D.P. (2000) Family size, infection and atopy: the first decade of the 'hygeine hypothesis'. *Thorax* **55** (suppl. 1), S2–10.

Stevenson, E.C., Turner, G., Heaney, L.G. *et al.* (1997) Bronchoalveolar lavage findings suggest two different forms of childhood asthma. *Clin. Exp. Allergy* **27**, 1027–35.

Stick, S., Arnott, J., Landau, L.I., Turner, D., Sy, S. and LeSoeuf, P. (1991) Bronchial responsiveness and lung function in recurrently wheezy infants. *Am. Rev. Respir. Dis.* **144**, 1012–15.

Stick, S.M., Burton, P.R., Gurrin, L., Sly, P.D. and LeSouef, P.N. (1996) Effects of maternal smoking during pregnancy and a family history of asthma on respiratory function in newborn infants. *Lancet* **348**, 1060–4.

Sulakvelidze, I., Inman, M.D., Rerecich, T. and O'Byrne, P.M. (1998) Increases in airway eosinophils and interleukin-5 with minimal broncho-constriction during repeated low-dose allergen challenge in atopic asthmatics. *Eur. Respir. J.* **11**, 821–7.

Tager, I.B., Hanrahan, J.P., Tostesan, T.D. *et al.* (1993) Lung function, pre- and post-natal smoke exposure, and wheezing in the first year of life. *Am. Rev. Respir. Dis.* **147**, 811–17.

Tasche, M.J.A., van der Wouden, J.C., Uijen, J.H.J.M. *et al.* (1997) Randomised placebo-controlled trial of inhaled sodium cromoglycate in 1–4 year old children with moderate asthma. *Lancet* **350**, 1060–4.

van Essen Zandvliet, E.E., Hughes, M.D., Waalkens, H.J. *et al.* (1992) Effects of 22 months of treatment with inhaled corticosteroids and/or beta-2 agonists on lung function, airway responsiveness, and symptoms in children with asthma. *Am. Rev. Respir. Dis.* **146**, 547–54.

van Essen Zandvliet, E.E., Hughes, M.D., Waalkens, H.J. *et al.* (1994) Remission of childhood asthma after long-term treatment with an inhaled corticosteroid (Budesonide): can it be achieved? *Eur. Respir. J.* **7**, 63–9.

Wildhaber, J.H., Devadason, S.G., Eber, E. *et al.* (1996) Effect of electrostatic charge, flow, delay and multiple actuations on the in vitro delivery of salbutamol from different small volume spacers for infants. *Thorax* **51**, 985–8.

Wilson, N., Sloper, K. and Silverman, M. (1995) Effects of continuous treatment with topical corticosteroids on episodic viral wheeze in preschool children. *Arch. Dis. Child.* **72**, 317–20.

Young, S., LeSouef, P.N., Geelhoed, G.C. *et al.* (1991) The influence of a family history of asthma and parental smoking on airway responsiveness in early infancy. *N. Engl. J. Med.* **324**, 1166–73.

Young, S., O'Keeffe, P.T., Arnot, J. and Landau, L. (1995) Lung function, airway responsiveness, and respiratory symptoms before and after bronchiolitis. *Arch. Dis. Child.* **72**, 16–24.

Chapter 8

Chung, K.F. (2000) Unmet needs in adult asthma. *Clin. Exp. Allergy* **30** (suppl. 1), 66–9.

Chung, K.F., Godard, P., Adelroth, E. *et al.* (1999) Difficult/therapy-resistant asthma: the need for an integrated approach to define clinical phenotypes, evaluate risk factors, understand pathophysiology and find novel therapies. ERS Task Force on Difficult/Therapy-Resistant Asthma. European Respiratory Society. *Eur. Respir. J.* **13**, 1198–208.

Drazen, J.M., Yandava, C.N., Dube, L. *et al.* (1999) Pharmacogenetic association between ALOX5 promoter genotype and the response to anti-asthma treatment. *Nat. Genet.* **22**, 168–70.

Israel, E., Drazen, J.M., Liggett, S.B. *et al.* (2000) The effect of polymorphisms of the beta(2)-adrenergic receptor on the response to regular use of albuterol in asthma. *Am. J. Respir. Crit. Care Med.* **162**, 75–80.

Kay, A.B. (2000) Overview of 'allergy and allergic diseases: with a view to the future'. *Br. Med. Bull.* **56**, 843–64.

Leckie, M.J., ten Brinke, A., Khan, J. *et al.* (2000) Effects of an interleukin-5 blocking monoclonal antibody on eosinophils, airway hyper-responsiveness, and the late asthmatic response. *Lancet* **356**, 2144–8.

Milgrom, H., Fick, R.B., Su, J.Q. *et al.* (1999) Treatment of allergic asthma with monoclonal anti-IgE antibody. rhuMAb-E25 Study Group. *N. Engl. J. Med.* **341**, 1966–73.

Rabe, K.F., Vermeire, P.A., Soriano, J.B. and Maier, W.C. (2000) Clinical management of asthma in 1999: the Asthma Insights and Reality in Europe (AIRE) study. *Eur. Respir. J.* **16**, 802–7.

Shirakawa, T., Enomoto, T., Shimazu, S. and Hopkin, J.M. (1997) The inverse association between tuberculin responses and atopic disorder. *Science* **275**, 77–9 [see comments].

Stirling, R.G. and Chung, K.F. (2000) New immunological approaches and cytokine targets in asthma and allergy. *Eur. Respir. J.* **16**, 1158–74.

Index

Accuhaler® 93–4
Acupuncture 88
Acute severe asthma 21, 107–13
  causes of 107–9
  clinical presentation 109–10
  management of 109, *Fig. 6.3*, *Fig. 6.4*
  pathology 107–8
  prevention of 109
  treatment of 110–13
  see also Exacerbation of asthma
Adenovirus 42
Adrenaline 113
Adult asthma 10–11, 21
  remission 11
Aeroallergens, avoidance of 100
  see also Pollen, Pollutants
Aggravating factors, *see* Risk factors
Air, cold 13, 76, 84, 86
  avoidance of 99
  hyperresponsiveness to 28
Airflow limitation
  causes of 58
  lung function measurements to assess 23–31
    expiratory reserve volume 24
    FEV_1 1–2, 23–6
    FVC 23–5
    inspiratory capacity 24
    lung volume 24
    MMEF 25–6
    PEFR 1, 16, 25–7
    tidal volume 24
    vital capacity 24
Airflow obstruction 1, 3, 16–18, 39
  diurnal variation 2
    monitoring 26–7
  effects of β agonists on 27
  effects of corticosteroids on 27
  symptoms 2
Airflow turbulence 16
Airway development 119

Airway epithelium
  cytokines produced by 49–50, 56
  transcription factors produced by 56
Airway hyperresponsiveness 54, 139
Airway inflammation 1–3, 22, 39, *Fig. 4.2*, 56–9, 63
  allergic 32
  cell counts of induced sputum 37
  corticosteroids suppress 63
  cytokines and 44–54
  exhaled nitric oxide 38
  investigation of 35–8
    fibreoptic bronchoscopy 36
    induced sputum 36–7
  ozone and 43
  T-helper cells and 44–6
Airway narrowing 59, 139
Airway obstruction 18–19, 54
Airway plugs, in acute severe asthma 108
Airway smooth muscle cells
  β_2-receptors 78
  cytokine production 54
  effect of bronchodilators on 78
  role in asthma 54–5, *Fig. 4.9*, 59
Airway smooth muscle hypertrophy 108
Airway wall oedema 58–9
  cysteinyl-leukotrienes and 76
  prevention by corticosteroids 63
  reduction by β-adrenergic agonists 78
Airway wall remodelling 54–5, *Fig. 4.8*, 121
  treatments aimed at 139
Airway wall thickening 108

Allergens
  aeroallergens, avoidance of 100
  Aspergillus fumigatus 20
  asthma exacerbations due to 31–2, 109
  bronchial constriction and 76
  bronchial hyperresponsiveness to 29
  cat 32, 42, 100, 145
  cockroach 33
  cytokine expression and 49–50
  dog 32
  early feeding with foreign proteins 41
  fungi 32–3
  house dust mite 10, 32, 41–2, 87, 100, 125
  mouse 33
  pets 41, 100, 125
  pollen 33, 41, 109
  risk factors 41–2, 109
  sensitization by 31, 41–2, 52, 119–20, 125–6
  see also Allergies, Risk factors
Allergic asthma 21
  anti-leukotriene therapy 76
  β-agonist therapy 84
  cytokines expressed in 49
  in the elderly 107–8
  nedocromil sodium therapy 74
  omalizumab and 142–3
  predisposition to 40–1, 52
  sensitization 119–20
  sodium cromoglycate therapy 74
  see also Allergies, Atopy, Exacerbations of asthma
Allergic bronchopulmonary aspergillosis 20–1
Allergic processes, regulated by action of IgE 52
Allergic rhinitis 28, 41, 87
  immunotherapy 88
  omalizumab and 142

Allergies 10, 13, 17, 31–3
  childhood asthma and 125–6
  diagnosis of 33
  food 33
  immunotherapy 87, 145
  improved hygiene and 46
  provocation tests 34–5
  serological tests 33–4
  skin-prick test 33
  T-helper imbalance and 45
  towards prevention of 144–5
  see also Allergens, Allergic
    asthma
Allopurinol 85
Alternaria 32–3
Alternative therapies 88–9
Aminophylline 85, 113
Ammi visnaga 88
Antibiotics, influence on asthma
  prevalence 46
Anticholinergic drugs 61, 78,
  86–8, 110, 140
  inhaled 103
  mode of action 86
  nebulized 86
  side-effects 87
Anti-flu vaccine 113
Antigen presentation, role of
  cytokines 49–50
Antihistamines 87, 122
Anti-IgE therapy 141–3
Anti-IL-4 therapy 141
Anti-IL-5 therapy 141
Anti-inflammatory drugs 101
  see also Corticosteroids,
    Theophylline
Anti-leukotrienes 75–7, 89, 103
  clinical use 76–7
  combined therapy with
    corticosteroids 76–7
  effect on PEFR *Fig. 5.6*
  mode of action 75–6
  side-effects 77
Aspergillus 33
Aspergillus fumigatus 20
Aspirin-induced asthma 13, 21,
  76, 100, 109, 138

Aspirin-induced
  bronchoconstriction 76
Asthma clinics 20, 96–7
Asthma Insights and Reality in
  Europe study 135
Asthma nurses 96
Asthma Quality of Life
  Questionnaire 31
Asthma syndrome 115, 127
Asthmatic bronchitis 18
Atopic asthma, *see* Allergic asthma
Atopy
  family order and 120
  genetic predisposition 40–1
  measles protects against 46
  parental 119
  T-helper imbalance in 45–6
  tuberculin hypersensitivity and
    46, 144
Auranofin 139
Autoimmune diseases 145

Bambuterol 81
BCG vaccination 144
Beclomethasone 65, 69–70, 72–3,
  75, 84, 93, 101, 103, 122
β-adrenergic agonists 1, 18, 61–2,
  66–7, 78–84, 89, 107, 109,
  138, 140
  administration of 81
  asthma deaths and 83
  chemical structure 79
  in childhood asthma 121
  choice of 81
  clinical use 79–81, 84
  effect on airflow obstruction 27
  effect on FEV_1 *Fig. 3.1*, 27
  inhaled *Table 5.2*, 110
  intravenous 113
  long-acting 79–81, 83, 103,
    128–9, 139
    combination with
      corticosteroids 81,
      Fig. 5.10, 83
  mode of action 78, *Fig. 5.8*
  nebulized route 79, 81, 84, 110,
    113

oral preparations 79, 81, 84
overreliance on 7
responders and non-responders
  145
safety studies 83–4
short-acting 101, 103, 106, 129,
  137
side-effects 83
tolerance to 83
β-blockers
  avoidance of 100
  exacerbations due to 107, 109,
    138
Blomia tropicalis 32
Bone densitometry 139
Bradykinin 58, 74
Breast feeding 41
British Thoracic Guidelines 3
Brittle asthma 13, 21, 138
Bronchial hyperresponsiveness
  1–3, 11, 17, 22, 28–31, 39,
  54, 58–9
  associated with high serum IgE
    41
  reduction of 31
    by corticosteroids 63
Bronchitis 1, 18
Bronchoconstriction
  cysteinyl-leukotrienes and 76
  inhibition by
    anti-leukotrienes 76
    nedocromil sodium 74
    sodium cromoglycate 74
  reversal by β-adrenergic agonists
    78
Bronchodilator drugs 1, 61–2,
  78–87, *Table 5.2*, 113
  intravenous 110
  reliance on 7
  response to 2
  treatment of childhood asthma
    126
  see also β-adrenergic agonists,
    Anticholingeric drugs,
    Theophylline
Bronchoscopy, fibreoptic 36,
  Fig. 4.2

Budesonide 65, *Fig. 5.4*, *Fig. 5.5*, 68–70, 72–3, 83, *Fig. 5.11*, 94, 101, 103, 122, 128

Cad1 32
Calcitonin-gene-related peptide 58
Candida 33
Carcinoid tumour 19
Cardiac arrythmias 86
Cardiac asthma 18
Cardiac dysrhythmias 83
Cataract 73, 122
Cellular interactions in asthma *Fig. 4.5*
c-Fos 56
Charcot–Leyden crystals 108
Chemokines 47–8
Chest tightness 13–14, 109
Childhood asthma 9–10, 21, 115–33
  administration of medications 124–5
  diagnosis 118, 126–7
  differential diagnosis 115–18
    congenital causes of wheeze 117
    cystic fibrosis 116, 118
    endobronchial foreign body 116–17
    Kartagener's syndrome 117
    oesophageal disease 117
    physical signs 116
    post-viral cough 115
    pulmonary oedema 118
  difficult asthma 132–3
  drug-delivery devices 130
  early exposure to allergens and 41–2
  environmental factors in 125–6
  growth suppression in 129–30
  investigations 123
  older children 127–33
    adherence to treatment 131
    exercise-induced asthma 129
    growth issues 129
    habit/honk cough 131–2

hyperventilation syndromes 132
  pharmacotherapy 128
  psychology 131–2
  vocal cord dysfunction 131
passive smoking and 42
persistence of 9–10
prophylactic medication 121
remission of 9–10
stress and 43
treatment of 121–6
  antihistamines 122
  β-adrenergic agonists 121
  corticosteroids 122
  cromolyns 122
  immunoglobulin 123
  ipratropium bromide 121
  salmeterol 123
  steroids 123
  steroid-sparing agent 123
  terbutaline 123
  theophylline 123
underdiagnosis of 14
viral respiratory infections and 42
Childhood infections, and T-helper cell imbalance 46
Chlorofluorocarbons 92–3
Chronic difficult asthma 138
Chronic obstructive pulmonary disease 3, 17–18
Chronic severe asthma 21, 138–9
Churg–Strauss syndrome 19, 21, 77
Cigarette smoking 7, 10–11, 17, 42–3, 85, 99, 107, 125
Cimetidine 85
Ciprofloxacin 85
Cladosporium 33
Classification of asthma 20–2
Clinical presentation 1–2, 13, 20–1, 109–10
Cockroach 33
Coffee 88
Cold air 13, 76, 84, 86
  avoidance of 99
  hyperresponsiveness to 28

Comorbidity factors, avoidance of 100
Compliance to therapy 131, 136
Computed tomography (CT) scan 18, 35
  of intrapulmonary airways *Fig. 3.8*
Congestive cardiac failure 18, 85
Conjunctivitis 5, 13, 87
Controlled breathing exercises 89
Corticosteroid-dependent asthma 21–2, 68, 138
Corticosteroid-resistant asthma 21–2, 138
Corticosteroids 7, 17, 19–20, 61–73, 89, 128
  clinical use 65–9
  combination therapy
    with long-acting β-adrenergic agonists 81, *Fig. 5.10*, 83, 135
    with theophylline *Fig. 5.11*
  effects on
    airflow obstruction 27–8, *Fig. 3.3*
    bronchial hyperresponsiveness 31
    inflammatory processes 66
    sputum eosinophilia 37
  first-pass metabolism in the liver 65, 69, 71
  inhaled 103, 107, 113, 128, 137–9, 144
    administration 68–9, 71
    benefits of 66
    clinical use 66
    currently available 69–71, *Table 5.1*
    dosage 66–7, 69
    early treatment with 66
    treatment of childhood asthma 122, 126
    pharmacokinetics 65, *Fig. 5.3*
    side-effects 71
  intravenous 69
  low-dose 101

Corticosteroids *cont.*
  mode of action 62–4, *Fig. 5.1*
  nebulized formulations 69, 104
  oral 69, 137–9
    in the elderly 108
    increased perinatal risks
        associated with 107
    side-effects 71, 73
  pharmacokinetics 64–5
  side-effects 71–3, 122
    adrenal suppression 72, 122
    alveolar underdevelopment
        123
    dermal thinning 73
    dysphonia 72
    effects on bone 72–3, 122
    effects on growth 73
    local 72
    oropharyngeal candidiasis 72
    skin bruising 73
    subcapsular cataract formation
        73, 122
    systemic 72–3
  structure 64, *Fig. 5.2*
  systemic 110
Corticosteroid-sparing agents 88,
    104, 123, 139
Cough 13, 16–17, 106, 109–10,
    115, 131–2
Cough-variant asthma 17, 21–2,
    126
Creola bodies 108
Curschmann's spiral 108
Cyclooxygenase-2 56, 58
Cyclosporin A 61, 88, 103, 123,
    133, 139
Cysteinyl-leukotrienes 52, 57,
    75–6, 145
  effects of *Fig. 4.10*, 76
  inhibition by anti-leukotrienes
    75–6
  synthesis 76
Cystic fibrosis 28–9, 116, 118
Cytokines 44–54
  antigen presentation 49–50
  airway wall remodelling and 54
  chemokines 47–8

expression in asthma 49,
    Fig. 4.5, 56
  corticosteroid suppression of
    63
  gene cluster 41
  growth factors 48–9
  lymphokines 47
  pollutants and 43
  pro-inflammatory cytokines 48
  promotion of 141
  role of 46–50
  suppression of 140–1

Datura stromanium 88
Death due to asthma 6–8, *Fig. 1.2*,
    Fig. 1.3, 21–3, 136
  exacerbations and 108
  excessive β-agonist use and 83
  reduction of 99
    associated with inhaled
        steroids 63, 99
  risk factors 6–7
  stress and 43
Definition of asthma 1–3
Dermal thinning 73
Dermatophagoides farinae 32
Dermatophagoides pteronyssinus 32
Desensitization 87
Diagnosis and assessment 13–22
  classification of asthma 20–2
  in the elderly 108
  physical examination 16
  questionnaires 13–14
  see also Differential diagnosis
Diclofenac 100
Diesel exhaust particles 43
Differential diagnosis 16–20
  allergic bronchopulmonary
        aspergillosis 20
  carcinoid tumour 19
  central airway obstruction 18
  in childhood asthma 115–18
  chronic obstructive pulmonary
        disease 17, 28, 35
  Churg–Strauss syndrome 19
  congestive heart failure 18
  pulmonary embolism 19

sarcoidosis 19, 29
  vocal cord dysfunction 19
Difficult-to-control asthma 137
Difficult-to-treat asthma 137–9
Diskhaler® 93
Disodium cromoglycate 122, 128
Diurnal variation
  airflow obstruction 2, 26–7
  PEFR 2, 17, 21, *Fig. 3.2*, 63
Drug delivery 89, 91
Dry-powder inhaler 68–9, 79, 81,
    89–90, *Fig. 5.12*, 93–4, 110,
    130
Dysphonia 72
Dyspnoea 18, 106
  see also Shortness of breath

East Germany, prevalence of
    asthma in 43
Eczema 13
Education 104–6
Elderly, asthma in the 107
Emphysema 1, 3, 17–18
Endobronchial foreign body
    116–17
Endothelin 55
Environmental risk factors 39–43,
    Fig. 4.1
  allergen exposure 41–2
  in childhood asthma 125–6
  chronic stress 43
  inhalable particulates 43
  ozone 43
  passive smoking 42, 99
  pollutants 43, 99–100, 126
  respiratory infections 13, 42,
    108
  respiratory irritants 43
  see also Allergens, Cold air
Eosinophilic bronchitis 17
Eosinophilic inflammation
    Fig. 4.7, 76
Eosinophils
  activation of 138
    IgE and 52
    inhibition of 74, 141
    associated cytokines 53–4

chemotaxis, cysteinyl-
leukotrienes and 76
cytokines produced by 49–50
nedocromil sodium, action on
74
platelet-activating factor
production by 58
production of 44, 47
inhibited by corticosteroids
63
sodium cromoglycate, action on
74
Eotaxin 48–9, 53–4, 63, 109
Ephedrine 88
Epidemiology of asthma 3–8
prevalence studies 3–5
see also Prevalence of asthma
Epidermal growth factor 48, 54
Epileptic fits 86
Episodic asthma 22
Erythromycin 85, 123
Europe, prevalence in 5, 135
Exacerbation of asthma 2, 13,
108–14
allergens and 31–2, 109
causes of 108–9
corticosteroid treatment and
Fig. 5.5, 69
drugs and 109
PEFR measurement of 27,
Fig. 3.2
predicting 109–10
profile of 15
stress and 43, 109
upper respiratory tract viral
infection and 42–3,
108–9
warning signs 106
see also Allergens, Allergies, Risk
factors
Exercise-induced asthma 13, 21,
29, Fig. 3.5, 76, 106
β-adrenergic agonists and 84, 99,
129
in children 129
corticosteroids prevent 63
hyperresponsiveness 2, 28–30

Fatal asthma 137
see also Death due to asthma
FcεRI receptors 41, 50, 52, 142
FcεRII receptors 51–2
Fel d1 32, 126
Fenoterol 81–2, 145
linked with asthma deaths 7,
83
Fibreoptic bronchoscopy 36,
Fig. 4.2
'Fixed' irreversible asthma 21–2
Flurbiprofen 100
Fluticasone propionate 65, 69–73,
83, 93, 103, 122
Food allergy 33, 126
Forced expiratory volume in 1
second (FEV$_1$) 1–2, 23–6
changes with age Fig. 1.4
changes with time Fig. 3.1
response to
allergen inhalation Fig. 3.7
anti-IL4 therapy 141
β-adrenergic agonists 27,
Fig. 5.9
bronchoconstrictors 29,
Fig. 3.4
corticosteroids 28
exercise 29
omalizumab 143
theophylline and budesonide,
Fig. 5.11
Forced vital capacity (FVC) 23–5
Formoterol Fig. 5.5, 79–3, 94,
103
duration of effect of 80

Gastro-oesophageal reflux 126,
138
GATA-3 56
Genetic factors
cytokine gene cluster 41
gene for
IgE receptor 41
interferon-γ 41
interleukin-4R 41
inheritance of atopy 40–1
linkage studies 41

maturation of cellular immune
function 45
susceptibility genes 40
twin studies 39–40
Genomic imprinting 41
Global Initiative for Asthma
Management and Prevention
95
Goblet cell hyperplasia 54
Gold salts 88, 139
Granulocyte/macrophage colony
stimulating factor 48–50, 53,
56, 63
Growth, effects of corticosteroid
therapy on 73
Growth factors 48–9, 54
Guidelines to the treatment of
asthma 95, 135

Health economics of asthma 8
impact of self-management on
105
Herbal medicines 88
Histamine
hyperresponsiveness to 2,
28–30, Fig. 3.4
release by mast cells 52
nedocromil sodium and 74
sodium cromoglycate and 74
role in asthma 56
Histamine H1 receptor antagonists,
as asthma treatment 56
Homeopathy 88–9
Hospital
admission to 5–7, 22, 110
asthma management in 96–7
discharge from 113
House dust mite 32, 41–2
reducing exposure to 100, 125
sensitivity to 10
immunotherapy for 87
Hydrocortisone 69, 110
Hygiene hypothesis 46
Hyperventilation syndromes 132
Hypnosis 89
Hypokalaemia 83
Hyposensitization 87

Precipitating factors 15, 31
  see also Risk factors
Prednisolone 27–9, 69, 102–3,
  110, 113
Pregnancy, asthma in 106–7
Premenstrual worsening of asthma
  138
Pressurized metered-dose inhaler
  91–3, 110
  breath actuated 92
  CFC-free 92–3
  manually actuated 91
  spacer devices 92
  see also Metered-dose inhaler
Prevalence of asthma
  East Germany 43
  European variation 5, 135
  increase in 5
  long-term allergen exposure and
    32
  UK 5, 135
  worldwide variation 4–5
Pro-inflammatory cytokines 48
Prostaglandins, potential role 58
Psychology of asthma 131–2
Pulmonary embolism 19
Pulmonary function tests, *see* Lung
  function tests
Pulmonary oedema 118

Quality-of-life scores 5, 31
Questionnaires
  for diagnosis and assessment
    13–14, 21
  random survey questionnaires
    5–6
Qvar® 93

RANTES 48–50, 56, 63, 109
Refractory asthma 137
Remission of asthma 9–11, 22,
  144
Reproterol 81–2
Respiratory irritants 43
Respiratory syncytial virus 42
Respiratory tract infections 13, 42,
  108

Rheumatoid arthritis 145
Rhinoconjunctivitis 5, 13
Rhinosinusitis 13, 100, 138
Rhinovirus 42, 108–9
Rifampicin 85
Risk factors 15, 39–43
  allergens 31–3, 41–2, 100, 109
    cat 32, 42, 100, 145
    cockroach 33
    dog 32
    early feeding with foreign
      proteins 41
    fungi 32–3
    house dust mite 10, 32, 41–2,
      87, 100, 125
    mouse 33
    pets 41, 100, 125
    pollen 33, 41, 109
    avoidance of 99, 100
  bronchial hyperresponsiveness
    29
  chronic stress 43
  cigarette smoking 7, 10–11, 17,
    42–3, 85, 99, 107, 125
  cold air 13, 76, 84, 86, 99
  environmental 39, 40–3, *Fig. 4.1*
  exercise 99
  genetic 39–41, *Fig. 4.1*
  inhalable particulates 43
  ozone 43, 99
  passive smoking 42, 99
  pollutants 43, 99–100, 127
  respiratory infections 13, 42,
    108
  respiratory irritants 43
Rotahaler® 93

Salbutamol 27, 79, 81–3, 93
Salmeterol 79–84, 93, 103, 123,
  128
  duration of effect of 80, *Fig. 5.9*
Sarcoidosis 19, 29
School nurses 96
Schools, asthma in 96
Seasonal asthma 13, 21
  antihistamines and 87
  Step-up treatments 104

Self-management 104–6
  plan 106, 113
Sensitization 10, 13
  by allergens 31, 41–2, 52, 125–6
Serological allergy tests 33–4
Severe therapy-resistant asthma
  137–9
Severity of asthma 5–6, 15–16,
  21–2, *Table 2.1*
Shortness of breath 13–14, 16, 18,
  106, 109
Skin bruising 73
Skin-prick tests, to common
  aeroallergens 33, *Fig. 3.6*
Smooth muscle hyperplasia 54
Sodium cromoglycate 61, 73–5,
  99, 102, 107, 129
  clinical use 75
  dosage 75
  mode of action 74
  pharmacokinetics 74
  side-effects 75
Spacer devices *Fig. 5.12*, 92, 124–5,
  130
Spinal manipulation 89
Spinhaler® 93
Sputum
  eosinophilia 37, 108
    suppression of 54
  induced for investigation of
    airways inflammation
    36–7, *Fig. 3.9*
  neutrophilia 108
Stem cell factor 52
Steroid-dependent asthma 137
  see also Corticosteroids
Steroid-resistant asthma 137
Steroid-sparing agents 88, 103,
  123, 139
Stress, and asthma exacerbations
  43, 109
  and onset of childhood asthma
    43
Subepithelial fibrosis 3, 54
Substance P 58
Sulphite-containing foods 100
Sulphur dioxide 74, 86, 99

Sulphur metabisulphite 74
Susceptibility genes 40
Sympathomimetics, *see*
β-adrenergic agonists
Symptomatic asthma 137

Tachycardia 83, 110
Teachers, role of 96
Terbutaline *Fig. 5.4*, 79, 81–2, 133
T-helper cell imbalance 45–6, 49,
51–2, 141, 144
T-helper cells 44–6
T-helper 1 45–7, 120
boosting 144–5
T-helper 2 45–7, 49, 120
involvement in airway wall
remodelling 54
T-helper progenitor 47
differentiation of *Fig. 4.3*
Theophylline 61, 67, 78, 84–6,
88, 103, 107, 123, 128, 139
clinical use 85
combination therapy with
corticosteroids *Fig. 5.11*
mode of action 84–5
pharmacokinetics 85
side-effects 84–6, 123

Therapy, new approaches to
139–41
Thromboxane, potential role in
asthma 58
Thunderstorms 109
Tiotropium bromide 86
Transcription factors 56
binding of corticosteroid
receptor complex to 63
blocking 141
Transforming growth factor β 48,
54
Treatment, delays in obtaining 23,
121
Trigger factors 13–14
see also Risk factors
Tuberculin, hypersensitivity to 46
Tumour necrosis factor 47–50,
53
Turbohaler® 93–4
Turbutaline 94
Twin studies 39–40

UK, prevalence in the 5
Underdiagnosis 14
Undertreatment 136
Urticaria 87

Vaccination, influence on asthma
prevalence 46
Vascular cell adhesion molecule-1
48, 53, 141
Ventolin® 93
Viral infection of upper respiratory
tract 10–11, 108
Vocal cord dysfunction 19, 131
Volume-spacer device 68, 72

Wheeze 1, 9, 13–14, 16, 18–19,
42, 84, 106, 110, 115–16
congenital causes of 117
history of intermittent 3
in infancy 118–20, 124, 127
airway development and
119
prognosis of 120
viral-associated 119–21
Worldwide variation of prevalence,
Fig. 1.1, 4–5
Worsening asthma, signs of 16

Yoga 89

Zafirlukast 76–7
Zileuton 76